Medicare Laboratory Payment Policy

Now and in the Future

Dianne Miller Wolman, Andrea L. Kalfoglou, and
Lauren LeRoy, Editors

Committee on Medicare Payment Methodology for
Clinical Laboratory Services

Division of Health Care Services

INSTITUTE OF MEDICINE

NATIONAL ACADEMY PRESS
Washington, D.C.

NATIONAL ACADEMY PRESS · 2101 Constitution Avenue, N.W. · Washington, D.C. 20418

NOTICE: The project that is the subject of this report was approved by the Governing Board of the National Research Council, whose members are drawn from the councils of the National Academy of Sciences, the National Academy of Engineering, and the Institute of Medicine. The members of the committee responsible for the report were chosen for their special competences and with regard for appropriate balance.

Support for this study was provided by the Health Care Financing Administration (Contract No. 500-99-0023).

International Standard Book No. 0-309-07266-2

Medicare Laboratory Payment Policy: Now and in the Future is available for sale from the National Academy Press, 2101 Constitution Avenue, N.W., Box 285, Washington, DC 20055. Call 800-624-6242 or 202-334-3938 (in the Washington metropolitan area), or visit the NAP online bookstore at www.nap.edu.

The full text of *Medicare Laboratory Payment Policy: Now and in the Future* is available on-line at www.nap.edu.

Printed in the United States of America.

The serpent has been a symbol of long life, healing, and knowledge among almost all cultures and religions since the beginning of recorded history. The image adopted as a logotype by the Institute of Medicine is based on a relief carving from ancient Greece, now held by the Staatliche Museen in Berlin.

"Knowing is not enough; we must apply.
Willing is not enough; we must do."
—Goethe

INSTITUTE OF MEDICINE

Shaping the Future for Health

THE NATIONAL ACADEMIES

National Academy of Sciences
National Academy of Engineering
Institute of Medicine
National Research Council

The **National Academy of Sciences** is a private, nonprofit, self-perpetuating society of distinguished scholars engaged in scientific and engineering research, dedicated to the furtherance of science and technology and to their use for the general welfare. Upon the authority of the charter granted to it by the Congress in 1863, the Academy has a mandate that requires it to advise the federal government on scientific and technical matters. Dr. Bruce M. Alberts is president of the National Academy of Sciences.

The **National Academy of Engineering** was established in 1964, under the charter of the National Academy of Sciences, as a parallel organization of outstanding engineers. It is autonomous in its administration and in the selection of its members, sharing with the National Academy of Sciences the responsibility for advising the federal government. The National Academy of Engineering also sponsors engineering programs aimed at meeting national needs, encourages education and research, and recognizes the superior achievements of engineers. Dr. William A. Wulf is president of the National Academy of Engineering.

The **Institute of Medicine** was established in 1970 by the National Academy of Sciences to secure the services of eminent members of appropriate professions in the examination of policy matters pertaining to the health of the public. The Institute acts under the responsibility given to the National Academy of Sciences by its congressional charter to be an adviser to the federal government and, upon its own initiative, to identify issues of medical care, research, and education. Dr. Kenneth I. Shine is president of the Institute of Medicine.

The **National Research Council** was organized by the National Academy of Sciences in 1916 to associate the broad community of science and technology with the Academy's purposes of furthering knowledge and advising the federal government. Functioning in accordance with general policies determined by the Academy, the Council has become the principal operating agency of both the National Academy of Sciences and the National Academy of Engineering in providing services to the government, the public, and the scientific and engineering communities. The Council is administered jointly by both Academies and the Institute of Medicine. Dr. Bruce M. Alberts and Dr. William A. Wulf are chairman and vice chairman, respectively, of the National Research Council.

COMMITTEE ON MEDICARE PAYMENT METHODOLOGY FOR CLINICAL LABORATORY SERVICES

LAUREN LEROY (*Chair*), President and Chief Executive Officer, Grantmakers In Health
HOWARD BAILIT, Professor, University of Connecticut Heath Center
CHRISTOPHER BLADEN, Independent Consultant
WILLIAM HSIAO, K.T. Li Professor of Economics, Harvard School of Public Health
WILLIAM KERR, Senior Vice President, The Hunter Group
J. STEPHEN KROGER, Chief Executive Officer, COLA
JOHN MATSEN, Professor Emeritus, University of Utah
STEPHEN T. MENNEMEYER, Professor, Health Care Organizations and Policy, University of Alabama at Birmingham
DAVID SMALLEY, Professor, College of Medicine, University of Tennessee-Memphis
EARL P. STEINBERG, Senior Vice President, Resolution Health Strategies, Inc.
BRUCE STEINWALD, Independent Consultant, Washington, D.C.
ELEANOR TRAVERS, National Clinical Advisor, Medical Cost Effectiveness, Department of Veterans Affairs Headquarters

Study Staff

DIANNE MILLER WOLMAN, Study Director
ANDREA L. KALFOGLOU, Program Officer
NICCI T. DOWD, Senior Project Assistant
KRYSTAL JONES-FOY, Senior Project Assistant

Auxiliary Staff

JANET M. CORRIGAN, Director, Division of Health Care Services
MIKE EDINGTON, Managing Editor
JENNIFER CANGCO, Financial Advisor

Consultants

KATIE MERRELL, University of Chicago
ZACHARY DYCKMAN, CHPS Consulting (Center for Health Policy Studies)
HENRY MILLER, CHPS Consulting (Center for Health Policy Studies)

Copy Editor

FLORENCE POILLON

REVIEWERS

This report has been reviewed in draft form by individuals chosen for their diverse perspectives and technical expertise, in accordance with procedures approved by the National Research Council's Report Review Committee. The purpose of this independent review is to provide candid and critical comments that will assist the Institute of Medicine in making its published report as sound as possible and to ensure that the report meets institutional standards for objectivity, evidence, and responsiveness to the study charge. The review comments and the draft manuscript remain confidential to protect the integrity of the deliberative process. The committee wishes to thank the following individuals for their participation in the review of this report:

M. DESMOND BURKE, Director of Laboratories, Weill Cornell Medical College, Director of Clinical Laboratories, New York Presbyterian Hospital
SHELIA G. DUNN, President and CEO, Quality America Incorporated
RAY GAMBINO, Executive Vice President and Chief Medical Officer Emeritus, Quest Diagnostics
TERRY HAMMONS, Senior Vice President for Research & Education, Medical Group Management Association
LOUISE B. RUSSELL, Research Professor of Economics, Institute for Health Care Policy, Rutgers, The State University of New Jersey

Although the reviewers listed above have provided many constructive comments and suggestions, they were not asked to endorse the conclusions or recommendations nor did they see the final draft of the report before its release. The review of this report was overseen by George D. Lundberg, Editor in Chief and Executive Vice President, Medscape, appointed by the Institute of Medicine, and Christopher A. Sims, Professor, Princeton University, Department of Economics, appointed by the National Research Council's Report Review Committee, who were responsible for making certain that an independent examination of this report was carried out in accordance with institutional procedures and that all review comments were carefully considered. Responsibility for the final contents of the report rests entirely with the authoring committee and the Institute of Medicine.

Preface

Laboratory tests play a major role in clinical care, providing practitioners with the tools to diagnose disease, treat illness, and monitor the condition of patients. Technological innovations have enhanced the scope, quality, and sophistication of laboratory services, to the very real benefit of health professionals and patients alike. With new scientific advances, laboratory tests are likely to play an even greater role in the coming years. Yet bringing these advances to patients depends not only on science and technology, but also on the policies we have in place to provide coverage and payment for laboratory tests.

As the largest payer for clinical laboratory services in the nation, Medicare covers inpatient and outpatient testing for the elderly and disabled. Its system of paying for outpatient laboratory tests, however, has remained largely unchanged since it was established in 1984. It is structured so that key decisions regarding coverage, payment, and medical necessity are sometimes made nationally and sometimes by local private contractors who administer the Medicare program across the country. Constraints on payments have led to a decline in actual Medicare expenditures for clinical laboratory tests, while those for most other medical services have continued to rise. Concerns about how well Medicare's payment method reflects current costs of laboratory testing and about the ability of the system to keep up with anticipated changes in technology prompted the Congress to direct the Health Care Financing Administration (HCFA) to commission this study.

HCFA asked the Institute of Medicine (IOM) to assess the current payment system and investigate options to improve it against a backdrop of changes in laboratory testing over the past 20 years and expectations for future innovation and use of laboratory services. The committee appointed by the IOM to carry out this study embraced the opportunity to assist HCFA and the Congress, but quickly recognized the complexity of its task.

Clinical laboratory tests are performed in a variety of settings, from physicians' offices to large, sophisticated regional facilities. Like other sectors of the health system, the laboratory industry has been buffeted by changes in the financing and delivery of medical services. Yet despite decreases in payment rates for laboratory services, this dynamic and resilient industry continues to grow. The committee found no simple way to characterize it. The committee was also surprised by the paucity of data on the clinical laboratory industry, its financial health, and the costs of performing laboratory tests. A profile emerged from the information that IOM staff and consultants gathered with the help of both industry and government experts, but the committee was often frustrated by the lack of evidence to corroborate its considered judgments.

Designing a payment system for medical services requires balancing the interests of Medicare beneficiaries, providers of clinical laboratory services, and taxpayers who help support the Medicare program. The committee was encouraged that beneficiary access to outpatient clinical laboratory services generally appears to be good. At the same time, the lack of data to measure the extent of distortions in current payments or to determine how well the system will absorb new technological changes in laboratory testing was a source of considerable concern. This study provided the opportunity both to systematically review what is known and to chart a course for reform. Based upon analysis of available information, the committee concluded that timely action can avoid serious problems in the future.

Guided by a set of goals for Medicare payment policy adopted early in its deliberations, the committee found both the need and the opportunity for improvements in the current payment system. It concluded that there is no basis for assuming that current payment levels accurately reflect the costs of providing laboratory services. Whatever distortions exist can provide incentives for inappropriate use of laboratory tests, making the creation of a more rational method of payment imperative. To build a system that will stand the test of time, however, requires improvements in the ways tests are approved for payment and described for billing purposes, as well as valued for payment.

This report sets out the committee's findings and recommendations for improvements in Medicare policy related to payment for outpatient clinical laboratory services. The committee was concerned that sustaining the current, outmoded payment method would ultimately have an adverse effect on beneficiary access to laboratory services. It considered concerns raised by the laboratory industry but was also struck by the comfort level many expressed with fundamental aspects of the existing payment method. This was good news, because it provided a clear path to improving the Medicare payment system—one that first simplifies the system by creating a single national fee schedule based on current national payment limits and then promptly begins a process of moving toward payment levels that more reasonably reflect the resources required to provide each laboratory test.

Through its recommendations, the committee seeks to reduce administrative complexity and ambiguity, foster more efficient and appropriate use of laboratory tests, and create a more open and understandable system for establishing payments. The committee favors processes that allow meaningful input by those who have a stake in the outcome of Medicare payment policy decisions. It sees such involvement as an important element in maintaining the credibility of the payment system. It also sets its sights on a system that can efficiently accommodate future progress in laboratory science and technology. The committee's recommendations are directed to both HCFA and the Congress, since both legislative and administrative actions would be necessary to implement them.

The committee could not have accomplished its goals without the excellent staff work of Dianne Wolman, study director, and Andrea Kalfoglou, program officer, in both informing our discussions and synthesizing the outcome of our deliberations. Their tireless efforts to bring useful information and structure to the committee's work enabled us to be both focused and productive. The staff and I greatly appreciate the commitment and hard work of the committee members. They openly shared their views, provided timely feedback on staff work, and made every effort to work toward consensus while respecting the differences among them.

Finally, this study was undertaken at a time of considerable uncertainty and potential. We have great expectations for scientific breakthroughs in the detection and treatment of disease. At the same time, we cannot foretell how continued changes in the financing and delivery of health care may affect the availability of new or existing services. It is incumbent upon us to prepare for the future by designing systems that can adapt as circumstances change. It is in this spirit that the committee offers its recommendations for improving Medicare payment for outpatient clinical laboratory services.

Lauren LeRoy, Ph.D.
Chair

Acknowledgments

During the course of the study, the committee and staff were assisted by many individuals who generously shared their expertise. In addition, many organizations, associations, and government agencies contributed to our understanding of the clinical laboratory industry, the professionals who work in it, and the public programs that regulate it. We especially want to thank those private organizations and federal agencies that presented testimony at the committee's open meetings and via its Web site: AdvaMed (formerly the Health Industry Manufacturers Association), the American Association of Bioanalysts, American Association for Clinical Chemistry, American Clinical Laboratory Association, American Medical Association, American Society for Clinical Laboratory Science, American Society for Microbiology, American Society of Clinical Pathologists, Clinical Laboratory Management Association, and College of American Pathologists, the Food and Drug Administration, Centers for Disease Control and Prevention, Office of the Inspector General, and our sponsor, the Health Care Financing Administration (HCFA).

HCFA made this study possible through both its financial support and the technical assistance it provided. HCFA's clinical laboratory payment methodology is not easy to understand; this study would have been impossible without HCFA's help. The project officer at HCFA, Anita Greenberg, Medicare Health Insurance Specialist, and Tom Gustafson, director of HCFA's Purchasing Policy Group, Center for Health Plans and Providers, greatly facilitated our data collection efforts. Many others at HCFA (see Appendix A) helped tremendously by answering our endless questions.

The committee was fortunate to have input from expert consultants. Katie Merrell, Center for Health Administration Studies, University of Chicago, provided a background paper on a "Framework for Describing and Assessing Policy Options," analyses of the impact of the National Limitation Amount (see Appendix B), and ongoing guidance and clear thinking on payment issues. She was ably assisted by Geri Brennan, University of Chicago. In addition, the Institute of Medicine (IOM) commissioned background papers from CHPS Consulting on "Recent Developments and Trends in the Clinical Laboratory Industry" and "Technology Trends in the Clinical Laboratory Industry." We thank Zachary Dyckman, who was assisted by Bonnie Bisol Cassidy and Sarah Grantham, for the preparation of these papers. Under the leadership of Henry Miller, CHPS Consulting also conducted surveys and research on costs of and payments for clinical laboratory services. The report of the payment study by Zachary Dyckman is included in Appendix C.

During preparation of this report we benefited from technical reviews of particular chapters by Medicare payment experts: George Greenberg, executive advisor, Office of the Assistant Secretary for Planning and Evaluation, Department of Health and Human Services; Peter Kazon, attorney, Mintz Levin; and Charlie Spalding, retired senior technical advisor, HCFA, currently senior functional analyst, Computer Sciences Corporation. We thank them for their comments and advice. We take sole responsibility for any remaining factual errors.

The committee also received assistance from several individuals at IOM. Janet Corrigan, director, Board on Health Care Services, provided guidance throughout the study. Linda Kilroy and Kim Thomas, Office of Contracts and Grants; Jennifer Cangco and Kay Harris, Office of Finance and Administration; Claudia Carl, Mike Edington, and Jennifer Otten, Office of Reports and Communication; Sally Stanfield, National Academy Press; and Michael Reilly, National Academy of Science intern, also provided strong support.

Because so many people gave willingly of their time and expertise to assist the committee and staff in our search for data and understanding, we have included their names in Appendix A.

Contents

TABLES, FIGURES, BOXES, AND EXHIBITS

Tables

Figures

Boxes

Exhibit

Medicare Laboratory Payment Policy

Summary

The Committee on Medicare Payment Methodology for Clinical Laboratory Services studied many aspects of the current Medicare payment system, conducted original research, and heard testimony from many organizations representing the varied interests of laboratories and laboratorians. From the perspective of the beneficiary, the system is working. The committee could find no evidence that Medicare beneficiaries have difficulty getting necessary laboratory services. From the perspective of the laboratory industry, the system should be working better, with fewer administrative delays, geographic inconsistencies, and claims denials. From the perspective of the committee, the current system includes irrationalities, which could exacerbate current problems and jeopardize beneficiary access in the future. Medicare needs a more timely and appropriate method for integrating the proliferation of new technologies anticipated in the near future and simpler, more transparent administrative procedures. To this end, the committee recommends that the Medicare program implement a single, national, rational fee schedule that reflects the resources used to produce the services, simplify and open its administrative procedures, and collect data to monitor and assess the impact of the recommended changes.

INTRODUCTION

Clinical laboratory tests are a key component of modern health care. Through the examination of body fluids and tissues, laboratory tests reveal important chemical and biological information about the body.[1] Laboratory tests represent a small share of health spending, but play a complementary and an integral role in good medical care. They help physicians to diagnose and treat patients. Technological changes in laboratory testing, both those currently in the pipeline and those anticipated in the near future, offer the prospect of new opportunities for diagnostic improvements. These changes, however, are often associated with expensive new laboratory tests and testing methodologies and will place an increasing burden on the payment system for timely, fair, and appropriate determinations of payment levels and medical necessity.

Medicare, the federal program providing coverage of health care services for the elderly and disabled, is the largest payer of clinical laboratory services. It pays 29 percent of the nation's laboratory bill for inpatient and outpatient services (Klipp, 2000). The Medicare Part B fee schedule for outpatient laboratory services accounts for approximately one-third of what Medicare spent for laboratory services, or 1.6 percent of its total annual budget, in 1998 (Gustafson, 2000).

Although outpatient clinical laboratory tests are only a small portion of the Medicare budget, Medicare payment policy for laboratory services is significant because it influences state Medicaid and private payers' policies and payment rates. Laboratory tests also influence health care expenditures far beyond their proportion of actual costs because decisions about the provision of other medical services often hinge on the results of laboratory tests.

Designed in the early 1980s, Medicare payment policy for outpatient laboratory services is now outdated. Payments are not consistently related to costs, and while payment rates have been modestly adjusted for inflation, neither the rates nor the basic payment methodology has evolved to take into account technology, market, and regulatory changes. Laboratory interest groups testified that the outdated payment system has created serious administrative and financial burdens for laboratories, although systematic evidence of major problems for patients, physicians, Medicare, or private insurers is lacking. Theoretically, when prices do not reflect costs, they have the potential to inappropriately influence clinical decision making, inhibit innovation, waste taxpayer dollars, and limit beneficiary access to care. In the case of clinical laboratory tests, the financial incentives of the physician ordering the test are not directly related to the financial incentives of the laboratory conducting the test and receiving payment for it; however, the physician's incentives could be subject to influence by the laboratories. Again, evidence of such effects is lacking.

Clinical laboratory testing is in the midst of major technological innovations, and regulatory and payment policies must be able to accommodate positive changes. The mapping of the human genome and other scientific advances

---

[1]Medicare covers clinical laboratory tests used to diagnose disease, screen patients to identify abnormalities, or monitor a patient's condition. It does not cover other laboratory services such as screening for drugs of abuse, conducting forensic investigation, evaluating a person's health for life insurance, and testing as a part of clinical research and drug development.

lead laboratory experts to expect major advances in clinical tests and methodologies in the near future, particularly in the areas of genetic testing, surface markers to identify specific types of cancers, pharmacogenomics to individualize drug treatments, and molecular-level tests. They foresee these diagnostic advances clearly; whether scientific advances for treatments will keep pace is less clear.

Recognizing the problems of the Medicare outpatient payment system for clinical laboratory services, Congress mandated that the Department of Health and Human Services (DHHS) arrange for the Institute of Medicine (IOM) of the National Academies to examine the laboratory industry, including environmental and technological trends; to collect data on costs and payments for certain laboratory tests if possible; to assess current Medicare payment policy; to evaluate payment policy alternatives, including costs and other aspects of implementation; and to make recommendations to improve the system (Balanced Budget Act of 1997 [BBA]; Public Law 105-33). The IOM was selected because its unique advisory process uses groups of independent, volunteer experts to analyze issues and make policy recommendations.

To conduct the study, the IOM formed a committee of 12 experts, including laboratorians, physicians, economists, health care administrators, and health policy analysts. The five committee meetings included open sessions for public testimony and data gathering. The IOM commissioned three background papers and a study on costs and payments for laboratory services. The committee focused on Medicare payment methodology, but related issues such as coverage policy and coding systems were also addressed. This summary highlights some of the key issues, conclusions, and recommendations from the full report.

THE LABORATORY INDUSTRY

In 1999, 170,102 clinical laboratories conducted 5.7 billion laboratory tests for both inpatients and outpatients in the United States (Tables 1 and 2).[2] Approximately $35 billion was spent on the provision of clinical laboratory services. Although overall health expenditures have continued to rise faster than growth in the gross domestic product in recent years (Wolf, 1999), total expenditures for laboratory services provided in all settings atypically have declined (Klipp, 2000).

Four main types of laboratories provide clinical laboratory services:

1. **Hospital-based laboratories:** Hospital-based laboratories conduct more tests than all other types of laboratories combined. In 1999, 8,560 hospital-based laboratories (Table 1) conducted almost 3 billion laboratory tests (Table 2), pro-

---

[2]Generally, when this report refers to the clinical laboratory industry, it includes the three types of laboratories discussed below: hospital-based, physician office, and independent laboratories. Other laboratories will be discussed, but they typically do not bill under the Medicare Part B outpatient system. When manufacturers of laboratory tests, equipment, and chemicals are included, this will be specified.

viding services for inpatients and outpatients and some community physicians. Many hospitals operate more than one laboratory. Independent laboratories run some hospital-based laboratories.

2. **Independent laboratories:** In 1999, 4,936 independent laboratories (Table 1) conducted 26 percent of laboratory tests in the United States, or 1.5 billion (Table 2), for physicians, hospitals, and other health care providers. These laboratories are often regional, serving large geographic areas, with single companies operating multiple laboratory facilities. Independent laboratories underwent rapid consolidation during the 1990s. Two large, multisite corporations now absorb more than half of the revenues of independent laboratories.

3. **Physician office laboratories:** Most of the 105,089 physician office laboratories (POLs) conduct a low volume of simple, inexpensive tests that provide immediate, on-site results to physicians (Table 1). Large, group practice POLs provide a range of tests at volumes comparable to those of local independent laboratories.

4. **Other laboratories:** Laboratory tests performed at end-stage renal disease centers, home health agencies, and nursing homes are frequently not paid out of the Medicare outpatient laboratory benefit. These "other laboratories" account for slightly more than 30 percent of all laboratory facilities (Table 1), but they conduct only 10 percent of all tests (Table 2).

Because the laboratory industry is so diverse and data describing it are so limited, it is difficult to draw definitive conclusions about trends. The industry has been characterized both by periods of growth and by a variety of constraints. Currently, test volume is up, but Medicare spending for outpatient laboratory services is down. The laboratory industry appears to be both resilient and adaptable, but also vulnerable to environmental trends. For instance, managed care and federal cost containment measures initially cut into laboratory profits, but the major national independent laboratories not only have survived, but have now rebounded financially. Hospital-based laboratories expanded their outpatient and outreach services in response to declines in inpatient laboratory de-

TABLE 1 Number of Laboratories by Type of Facility, 1999–Early 2000

Type of Facility	Number of Laboratories	Percentage of Total
Hospital laboratories	8,560	5
Independent laboratories	4,936	3
Physician office laboratories	105,089	62
Other	51,517	30
Total	170,102	

SOURCE: Health Care Financing Administration, 2000.

TABLE 2 Test Volume by Type of Facility, 1999–Early 2000

Type of Facility	Volume (millions)	Percentage of Total
Hospital laboratories	2,958.2	52
Independent laboratories	1,514.2	26
Physician office laboratories	656.4	11
Other	597.1	10
Total	5,725.9	

NOTE: Volume figures include both inpatient and outpatient tests performed for all public and private sector payers.

SOURCE: Health Care Financing Administration, 2000.

mand to the point where their market share is growing. The numbers of POLs declined in the late 1980s in reaction to federal regulatory policies, but they are now increasing, partially in response to an increase in the number of tests that can be conducted simply.

Many factors affect the cost of providing laboratory services. New regulatory requirements increased costs for some laboratories; however the industry has also reduced costs through consolidation, automation, and other innovations that have simplified testing and administrative procedures. Future innovation in automation, test methodology, and information technology will require substantial investment but should also increase efficiency. More complex testing, particularly genetic testing, may routinely require specialized expertise to interpret the findings for the ordering clinician which will add to the cost of providing the test.

The overall quality of laboratory testing is improving. Experts speculate on a number of technological-, regulatory-, and professional-related reasons. Portable testing equipment makes it easier to test patients at the bedside or during a visit to the doctor. In addition to convenience, testing closer to the patient leads to faster results that may facilitate diagnosis and treatment. Improvements in quality are seen in improved proficiency test results and fewer deficiencies during on-site inspections. Payment trends have the potential to affect beneficiary access to laboratory testing, although there is no evidence that they have done so. The lack of appropriate billing codes, Medicare coverage decisions, and payment barriers could delay beneficiary access to new technology. If it becomes more difficult to absorb reduced payments, the industry might no longer offer tests when costs exceed payments.

THE CURRENT MEDICARE PAYMENT SYSTEM

Medicare currently pays for outpatient clinical laboratory tests using a prospective payment system (PPS) established in 1984 and based on 1983 charge data. The amount of payment is known before a service is delivered. Payments for 1,100 tests are set separately in fee schedules for each of 56 geographic jurisdictions, limited by national fee caps called National Limitation Amounts (NLAs). Payments are based on what laboratories charged in 1983, updated periodically for inflation. Laboratories accept Medicare fees as full payment—there is no beneficiary cost sharing. The Health Care Financing Administration (HCFA), the branch within DHHS that administers the Medicare program, and private contractors to HCFA known as carriers and fiscal intermediaries (FIs),[3] make and interpret policy, set prices, and process claims.

Most general policy decisions guiding program operations are made at the national level by HCFA within the constraints of congressionally set authority. Medicare contractors process and pay claims from laboratories. Traditionally, carriers have taken responsibility for developing local coverage policies that determine when particular tests are medically necessary and for calculating the local fee schedules, but some of this responsibility has shifted back to HCFA's central office in recent years. Contractors review claims and may deny payment if they determine the service was not medically necessary in a particular case. There are inescapable inconsistencies in this process. Decisions about how much to pay for new tests are made both by the carriers and by HCFA. The payment system, thus, is complicated by the fact that decisions about both coverage and payment are made in each of the 56 distinct jurisdictions.

GOALS FOR A PAYMENT SYSTEM

To meet its charge, the committee first defined the goals that should guide payment policy. The following five goals are broadly applicable to the Medicare payment system and are specifically relevant to payments for outpatient clinical laboratory services.

1. **Beneficiary access:** All Medicare beneficiaries should have access to appropriate services on a timely basis. Financial barriers should not limit beneficiary access to appropriate services. When it is medically appropriate, testing ought to be expedited.

2. **Flexibility:** The payment methodology should have formal mechanisms to promptly recognize and determine payment for newly approved technology, to adjust payment levels when necessary, and to update payment amounts in

---

[3]HCFA's contractors include carriers, which process laboratory claims from POLs and independent laboratories, and FIs, which process claims from hospital-based and other institutional laboratories.

response to scientific and economic shifts in the health care environment that affect the costs of producing laboratory services.

3. **Transparency:** The process for setting payment amounts and payment policies should be understandable and open to input from the public and providers.

4. **Value:** Value encompasses the efficient production and appropriate use of laboratory services, as well as minimizing fraud, waste, and abuse. The goal is to produce a positive health outcome for the beneficiary using high-quality, appropriate health care services.

5. **Administrative simplicity and efficiency:** The payment system should strive for simplicity and efficiency in its administrative operations for the provider, payer, and patient.

ASSESSMENT OF THE CURRENT MEDICARE PAYMENT SYSTEM

The committee conducted an extensive examination of the Medicare payment system for outpatient laboratory services and assessed the current methodology in light of the committee's goals.[4]

- **Beneficiary access:** The committee found no evidence that beneficiaries have difficulty obtaining outpatient clinical laboratory services. The current geographic locations, number of sites, and capacity of the laboratories generally provide adequate access for beneficiaries. The Medicare program imposes no financial barriers to outpatient clinical laboratory services for beneficiaries. Finally, the committee found no evidence that Medicare beneficiaries are being denied STAT (literally, at once) tests when medically indicated.
- **Flexibility:** The committee concluded that existing mechanisms for keeping payments up to date are inadequate. The inflation factor and the NLA level raise or lower fees across the board for all tests and do not provide adjustments to accommodate changes needed in payment levels for specific tests. The process for integrating new technologies into the payment system, including determinations of coverage, assignment of billing codes, and development of appropriate prices, is slow, administratively inefficient, and closed to stakeholder participation. These problems are likely to become increasingly important with the anticipated changes in laboratory technology and medical practice.
- **Transparency:** The committee concluded that the current payment system lacks "openness" and adequate procedures for stakeholder involvement. Clear and consistent information on how the system works and opportunities for the public and stakeholders to have input into decision processes are limited.
- **Value:** The committee found it had little data with which to judge whether Medicare spending in aggregate is too high or low, whether Medicare is

---

[4]The examination included interviews with many HCFA staff, other stakeholders, and laboratory services and financing experts; testimony from industry associations; and a review of relevant program-related documents, data, and studies.

paying reasonable amounts for individual tests and services, or whether physicians are ordering tests appropriately. The committee concluded that Medicare purchases tests that meet Medicare standards for its beneficiaries with minimal or no beneficiary access problems. Medicare payment rates appear to be within the range of private payments (Appendix C).

• **Administrative simplicity and efficiency:** The committee concluded that administration of the Medicare outpatient laboratory payment system, with its 56 separate fee schedules and 56 separate processes for coverage determination, is unnecessarily complex and inefficient, particularly in the way the system incorporates new technologies and determines whether or not a laboratory's claim should be paid. Since most of the fees on the 56 separate fee schedules are close to the NLA, this complexity is unnecessary.

RECOMMENDATIONS

After analysis of the current payment method and alternative policies, the committee reached consensus on 12 recommendations for improving Medicare's payment system for outpatient clinical laboratory services. The committee's choices were guided by its previously stated goals for an ideal payment system. The committee considered the administrative, legislative, and financial steps necessary to implement alternative payment methods. The committee's recommendations provide broad, general policy guidance. The details regarding how recommendations are implemented could have a significant impact on ultimate implementation costs.

The first six recommendations are interrelated and cascade from the first recommendation, which broadly defines the preferred payment system and flows into more detailed recommendations concerning specific elements of the system and its implementation. The first six recommendations focus specifically on payment methodology. They address issues such as how to establish the relative value of one test versus another and how to determine the relative resource use of different tests. They do not conclude whether current Medicare aggregate payments or the payment for a particular test is too high or too low.

The final six recommendations focus on problems in the current system. These recommendations can be implemented independently or concurrently with the first six. They consider such issues as the structure of the claims-processing contractors and how to improve payment-related administrative procedures.

Because changes in the current Medicare payment formula could require new legislation, implementation of many of the committee's recommendations will entail congressional action. The committee recommends that HCFA, the administration, and the Congress work together to develop the necessary enabling authority and funding.

RECOMMENDATION 1: Medicare payments for outpatient clinical laboratory services should be based on a single, rational, national fee schedule.

In effect, there is already a national fee schedule, since most services are paid at the National Limitation Amounts. Maintaining a system of 56 fee schedules that, in the vast majority of cases, pays a single, national fee is confusing to stakeholders and increases the burden of administering the system. A national fee schedule means a single set of payments for all outpatient clinical laboratory services, with adjustments for differences in local labor costs, prices for goods and services the laboratory purchases, and other relevant factors.

The long-term goal of a national fee schedule is to establish relative payment amounts that accurately reflect the relative resource requirements of providing services, minimizing the financial incentives to overuse or underuse services. In other words, if Test A for one condition generally costs laboratories twice as much to produce as Test B for another condition, the payment for Test A should be twice as much as for Test B.

The committee considers this important for promoting the clinically appropriate use of laboratory services and ensuring that beneficiaries continue to have access to services. The key building blocks of such a fee schedule include (1) a relative value scale; (2) a dollar conversion factor that translates the relative values into payment amounts; (3) any adjustments for laboratory, beneficiary, or other characteristics, such as geographic location; and (4) a mechanism for periodic updates. HCFA has extensive experience establishing relative values, fee schedule payment adjustments, and update mechanisms, particularly with the physician payment methodology.

Moving to a single national fee schedule is a logical first step because it will make it easier to develop refined, resource-based relative payment amounts, will simplify the system, and will reduce some administrative complexities and inconsistencies. The committee makes additional, specific recommendations about how to move quickly to a national fee schedule and then recommends a process for refining and improving it.

RECOMMENDATION 2: On an interim basis, relative payments for Medicare outpatient clinical laboratory services should be based on the current National Limitation Amounts.

The NLAs are an appropriate starting point for the national fee schedule, but HCFA should move quickly to refine them. Moving to a national fee schedule based on the NLAs formalizes current, de facto Medicare outpatient laboratory payments. Use of the NLAs as a starting point should minimize dislocations and disruptions for laboratories, beneficiaries, and contractors.

The committee does not make a recommendation on whether aggregate spending on clinical laboratory services ought to be increased or decreased, and it recognizes that projected spending levels are often an outcome of the budget process. The committee notes, however, that under current law, Medicare outpatient clinical laboratory fees will not increase or decrease through 2002. If Congress and HCFA were to maintain this requirement while implementing the new fee schedule (i.e., projected aggregate outpatient clinical laboratory spending remains the same), then current NLA levels would have to be slightly reduced to permit the few carrier fees currently below the NLAs to rise. A preliminary analysis suggests that a reduction of the NLAs by as little as 1 or 2 percentage points may be sufficient to maintain the current level of aggregate spending (Appendix B). If a more detailed study shows that larger reductions in the NLAs would be needed if Congress were to call for maintaining budget neutrality, then the new fee schedule should be phased in over two or more years to minimize disruptions.

RECOMMENDATION 3: A data-driven consensus process for refining the new Medicare national fee schedule for outpatient clinical laboratory services should be developed. HCFA should explore alternative methods for gathering data to be used in the process.

The committee believes that a data-driven consensus approach is most likely to be a practical and successful approach to refining the fee schedule. Several interdisciplinary groups, which include experts and stakeholders such as laboratorians and HCFA policymakers, could both review and refine the NLA-based fee schedule or develop a completely new set of relative values. The groups, using data from many sources, could focus on every test or groups of similar tests, selected fees that are noticeably out of line, or those tests that contribute most to Medicare spending.

HCFA should examine the costs, potential value, strengths, and weaknesses of other approaches and methods for gathering data on costs and developing national relative values before refining or replacing the NLA-based fee schedule. The committee considered a number of approaches for establishing a relative value scale or relative payment rates.[5] These approaches are not mutually exclusive and could be combined in various ways to refine the NLA. Four approaches merit further consideration. Each option has specific risks, potential disruptions, and different consequences, depending on how it is designed. The potential impact of each approach should be examined to determine whether some adjustment might be desirable to mute the risk of a negative impact on beneficiary access or on the practice of medicine.

1. **Micro-costing studies:** HCFA would collect objective cost data related to specific services from laboratories, manufacturers, and other appropriate sources. The costs would include labor, equipment, supplies, transportation, and administrative functions such as regulatory compliance associated with the production of laboratory tests. The research could range from detailed cost studies of all laboratory services in a sample of all laboratories to targeted studies of selected tests and laboratories.

---

[5]The committee recognizes that setting the right prices is a necessary factor, but not sufficient to ensure cost-effective, medically appropriate treatment in every case.

2. **Competitive bidding demonstration:** HCFA would solicit bids on a specified list of tests from laboratories in a selected service area. Submitted bids should reveal costs of production, and, therefore, could be used as the basis for establishing relative values.

3. **Negotiated fee demonstration:** A demonstration in selected areas, based on a private sector model of negotiation, could be used by carriers and area laboratories to agree on a fee schedule. Like competitive bidding, this approach also provides a basis for developing national relative values.

4. **Charges:** The charges employed by laboratories on each Medicare claim could contribute to the development of relative values. However, because of uncertainty about how closely current charges reflect costs, this option could be used initially in conjunction with another approach to evaluate the nature of the relationship between charges and costs.

> **RECOMMENDATION 4: Medicare national fees for outpatient clinical laboratory services should be adjusted for geographic location. HCFA should also evaluate the need to adjust for certain other circumstances, particularly those likely to affect beneficiary access, and make recommendations to the Congress.**

Some costs, primarily labor and specimen transportation costs, may vary widely across the nation and between urban and rural areas, and would require an adjustment, as is made under most other Medicare payment methodologies. The committee does not support payment adjustments based on broad categories of laboratories, such as physician office, hospital-based, or independent laboratories; however, it is concerned that there may be situations in which lack of adjustment to national fees could affect beneficiaries' ability to obtain needed services. The committee recommends that HCFA study whether adjustments for differences in costs may be desirable for the following:

- **Qualified laboratories in sole community hospitals:**[6] These providers currently receive slightly higher Medicare outpatient laboratory payments. HCFA should study the implications for sole community hospitals of a new national fee schedule.
- **STAT tests:** The committee recognized that tests that must be conducted immediately for urgent or emergency care may present additional costs, but it could find no data to document a cost differential. If there is a need to recognize STAT tests in Medicare payments, care should be taken with the way in which

---

[6]A sole community hospital is located at least 25–35 miles from similar hospitals, serves at least 75 percent of the local residents needing such inpatient care, and meets the detailed criteria contained in 42 C.F.R. 412.92. To be a "qualified laboratory" in a sole community hospital, the laboratory must provide clinical diagnostic tests 24 hours a day, seven days a week, in order to serve the hospital's emergency room.

STAT circumstances are defined and their use should be monitored in order to minimize inappropriate use of the STAT designation.

RECOMMENDATION 5: Processes should be put in place to refine and periodically update the fee schedule for Medicare outpatient clinical laboratory services.

To remain viable, the fee schedule must respond to economic and scientific changes that affect the cost of providing services. Processes to refine and periodically update the fee schedule should include opportunities for industry and public input, review, and challenge. These procedures may vary for the different elements or building blocks of the fee schedule.

- **Update factor:** The update or conversion factor could be applied across the board to the current NLAs or to a fee schedule that is based on relative values. The process for updating the fee schedule should identify the responsible parties, the schedule for acquiring and analyzing data, and the factors that should be considered in developing the updated amount. Because the update factor will affect federal spending, it is likely to be established through the annual budget process. Although HCFA would ultimately be responsible for implementing updated rates, it might be appropriate to require the Medicare Payment Advisory Commission (MedPAC) or another suitable government agency to make recommendations to the Congress about the update factor.
- **Payment adjustments:** Review and revision of any geographic and other payment adjustments should include analyses of their likely effect on beneficiary access to laboratory services.
- **Relative values:** Periodic review of the relative values, however they were originally established, is essential for maintaining the integrity of the payment methodology.

RECOMMENDATION 6: To incorporate new tests into the Medicare laboratory fee schedule, there should be an open, timely, and accessible process that is subject to challenge. The process and fees produced should not impede clinical decision making that is essential to providing appropriate care.

The committee concluded that a consistent, public process for developing interim values for new laboratory services is essential for an effective payment system. HCFA should create a committee of laboratorians, pathologists, other physicians and scientific experts, health care policymakers, and economists to advise on setting interim relative values or national fees for new technologies. After interim relative values or fees for new services have been established, Medicare should allow time for diffusion of the new technology and stabilization of costs. The interim relative values for these new services should be reviewed and revised as necessary. Once they are "official," these services would be included in the periodic review of relative values for the full fee schedule.

RECOMMENDATION 7: HCFA should review alternatives to the current system for coding outpatient clinical laboratory services for claims processing. More accurate, open, and timely coding processes for new technologies as well as tests and services should be sought.

The committee heard testimony from several sources that the application process for a new Current Procedural Terminology (CPT) code[7] often adds to the time required to incorporate new technologies into the Medicare laboratory payment system. There are also problems with the inadequate specificity of the codes. Coding, the Medicare coverage process, and payment determinations are closely intertwined; tend to lack transparency; and can add considerably to the time required to incorporate a new test, new equipment, or a new testing methodology. The rapid development of anticipated new technologies will exacerbate this problem. HCFA should examine how to reduce coding delays within the current system and should explore alternative coding systems.

RECOMMENDATION 8: The current policy of not requiring beneficiary cost sharing for Medicare outpatient clinical laboratory services should continue. Cost sharing is unlikely to significantly reduce overuse or increase the detection of fraud and abuse; it could create barriers to access for the most vulnerable Medicare beneficiaries; and it would be financially and administratively burdensome for laboratories, patients, and the Medicare program depending on its design.

The committee recognizes the arguments supporting cost sharing elsewhere in the Medicare program. For laboratory services, however, the normal incentives of cost sharing are weakened because the patient does not initiate the use of laboratory services, usually has no contact with the laboratory, often has supplemental insurance that mutes the cost impact, and is unlikely to challenge the physician's order. Cost sharing is also unlikely to lead beneficiaries to detect fraud and abuse. Cost sharing could create a barrier to appropriate use of laboratory services for chronically ill and financially disadvantaged beneficiaries, which could ultimately lead to greater program costs if deferred testing delays diagnosis and leads to more costly treatment. Finally, administering copayments is impractical because the cost to the laboratory of billing and collecting the copayment will often exceed the expected payment amount.[8]

---

[7]The physicians' coding system, called Current Procedural Terminology, Fourth Edition (CPT-4), is maintained by the American Medical Association.

[8]A copayment of 20 percent would be less than $2.30 on average for the 100 highest dollar volume tests. The average number of tests per patient claim in some laboratories is

RECOMMENDATION 9: HCFA should discontinue use of International Classification of Diseases, Ninth Revision (ICD-9) diagnosis codes as the basis for determining the medical necessity of clinical laboratory tests. HCFA should assess the need for any approach to evaluating the medical necessity of individual laboratory tests prior to payment of a claim. In addition, HCFA should evaluate alternative approaches for identifying and reducing unnecessary or inappropriate laboratory testing.

Determinations of medical necessity based on diagnosis codes were instituted to improve the appropriateness of testing and, in part, to discourage fraud and abuse related to physician self-referral. Since implementation of the Stark legislation,[9] there has been less financial incentive for physicians to order unnecessary tests. In addition, experience has shown that the use of ICD-9 codes is not a sound basis for making judgments regarding the medical necessity of particular laboratory tests in specific patients.[10] One of the fundamental problems with the approach that the contractors currently use to make a determination of the medical necessity of a particular laboratory test for a particular beneficiary at a particular time is that, in many circumstances, it is likely to give the wrong answer. Moreover, the current system is easily gamed, is administratively burdensome, and does not place sufficient responsibility on the physician.

HCFA has developed a complex system of guidelines, some local and some national, including policies for 23 common tests, that advise physicians on what diagnosis codes constitute appropriate use of particular tests. The national policies for these 23 tests, recently developed under a negotiated rulemaking process (Neg Reg), are a considerable improvement over the many conflicting local medical review policies (LMRPs) that were in existence. The Neg Reg initiative, however, did not consider the underlying question of whether ICD-9 codes are a sound basis for determining medical necessity. The current system, although commendable in its intentions, is not effective in accomplishing its purpose. It creates a substantial administrative burden on laboratories and physicians, and the need for Medicare and its contractors to develop medical review policies to guide payment determinations.

HCFA currently can document neither the extent nor the nature of medically unnecessary testing. HCFA should monitor laboratory test trends to identify increases in unnecessary tests if they occur. As a prudent buyer, HCFA should examine a number of other approaches for promoting clinically appropriate use of laboratory tests including the following:

2.5, but the cost of producing and sending a letter could be more than $5.00. There would also be costs from bad debts.

[9]Under this legislation, physicians may not refer their patients to laboratories in which they or their family members have a financial interest.

[10]The code ICD-9 is a five-digit number indicating the diagnosis or symptoms of a patient.

• inclusion of outpatient clinical laboratory tests in the peer review organizations' (PROs') next scope of work;

• focused medical reviews of both prepayment and post payment, by contractors or PROs;

• development of approaches for identifying the inappropriate use of laboratory tests supported by the Agency for Healthcare Research and Quality (AHRQ);

• development of methods for holding physicians financially accountable for claims determined to be medically unnecessary; and

• creation of methods to detect and address fraud and abuse developed in conjunction with with the Office of the Inspector General (OIG).

RECOMMENDATION 10: In its policy formulation processes, HCFA should provide opportunities for stakeholder input and develop better communication with contractors and other stakeholders when policies are being developed and once they are adopted.

Many laboratory industry concerns about the Medicare payment system have their origins in the current lack of public input and the inadequate communication of policy decisions. Providers are more likely to accept Medicare payment policies, and accurately apply them, if they understand them and have the opportunity to participate in their development.

RECOMMENDATION 11: HCFA should move promptly to consolidate the number of contractors processing all Medicare outpatient clinical laboratory claims, including claims from physician office laboratories (POLs) and hospital-based laboratories. The design of this consolidation should ensure that claims processing by regional laboratory carriers will not require major new billing procedures for POLs or hospital-based laboratories. Efforts should be made to strengthen local provider services and relations between carriers and laboratories.

The committee believes that the standardization of program operations is an important aspect of the goal of administrative simplicity and efficiency. Thus, it supports the 1997 Balanced Budget Act mandate for the consolidation of clinical laboratory claims processors into four or five regional carriers and the designation of one carrier as the central statistical resource, and it encourages HCFA to implement this. The committee found that the current system of 56 carrier regions, with approximately 23 distinct carriers and 30 fiscal intermediaries, creates inconsistencies in the interpretation of HCFA policy and procedures, duplicates the cost of pricing new tests, and leads to variable interpretations of medical necessity for the same tests. Although it supports the standardization and consolidation of carriers, the committee recognizes the need for providers to have easy access to a contact within the carrier who understands the local health care environment and can provide the necessary advice and service.[11] Given the scope of this mandated change and the number of design issues yet to be decided, the committee cautions HCFA to monitor this change closely and beware of unintended consequences.

RECOMMENDATION 12: HCFA should collect the data needed to effectively manage the performance of the Medicare outpatient clinical laboratory payment system.

HCFA should collect baseline data to inform future policy considerations and additional data to measure the impact of policies, particularly on beneficiary access to care and on the diffusion of new technologies. Objectives and illustrative examples of baseline and performance measures related to the payment system goals set out by the committee include the following:

- **Beneficiary access**—*Objective:* Determine whether beneficiaries and physicians have adequate access to laboratory services. Possible measures include a sample survey of beneficiaries and physicians to obtain their assessment of any access problems and tracking changes in the number and distribution of laboratories participating in Medicare.
- **Flexibility**—*Objective:* Determine the effectiveness of methods to assign payments for new tests, adjust unreasonable fees, and update payment amounts. Possible measures include a comparison of Medicare and private payments for a broad sample of tests and health plans and tracking the average time needed to adjust unreasonable fees once the have been identified.
- **Transparency**—*Objective:* Determine how well stakeholders understand the processes for setting payment policies and their perceived ability to influence policies. Possible measures include a sample survey of laboratorians, carriers, and physicians to assess their knowledge and perceptions of HCFA's policy processes.
- **Value**—*Objective:* Determine the quality and cost of outpatient laboratory tests purchased by Medicare. Possible measures include monitoring Clinical Laboratory Improvement Amendments (CLIA) certification and performance status and claims denial rates, reasons for the denials, and the percentage of claims ultimately paid.
- **Administrative simplicity and efficiency**—*Objective:* Determine how well the key payment processes work within HCFA and in a sample of laboratories, physician practices, and contractors. Possible measures include a comparison among contractors of basic internal processes to assess their relative efficiency.

---

[11]In this report, the term "provider" generally refers to any individual or organization, such as a physician, laboratory, or hospital that provides care for Medicare beneficiaries. When reference to only one type of provider is intended, it will be specified.

CONCLUSION

Congress and HCFA have the opportunity to fix the current payment system for clinical laboratory services averting the possibility of a crisis in the future. Payments for some individual tests likely do not reflect the cost of providing services, and anticipated advances in laboratory technology will exacerbate the flaws in the current system. Problems with the outdated payment system could threaten beneficiary access to care and the use of enhanced testing methodologies in the future, although the committee found no evidence of this now. Although radical changes are not called for at this time, implementing the committee's recommendations will likely improve the efficiency of the system and ensure that Medicare beneficiaries continue to have access to high-quality laboratory services.

REFERENCES

Dyckman, Z., and B. B. Cassidy. 2000. *Recent Developments and Trends in the Clinical Laboratory Industry* (unpublished). Columbia, MD.

Gustafson, T. January 20, 2000. Testimony before the IOM Committee on Medicare Payment Methodology for Clinical Laboratory Services. Washington, DC.

Health Care Financing Administration (HCFA). March 2000 CLIA Provider Files.

Klipp, J. 2000. *Lab Industry Strategic Outlook 2000: Market Trends and Analysis.* Washington, DC: Washington G-2 Reports.

Merrill Lynch. 1999. *Quest Diagnostics: Leader in Sector with Improving Fundamentals.* reference # 60126501. New York, NY: Merrill Lynch.

Wolf, L. F. 1999. *Medicare and Medicaid Statistical Supplement in Health Care Financing Review.* Baltimore, MD: Office of Strategic Planning, Health Care Financing Administration.

1

Introduction

ORIGINS OF THIS STUDY

Clinical laboratory services represent a small proportion of total expenditures for medical services. In Medicare, payments for outpatient clinical laboratory tests account for only 1.6 percent of program spending (Gustafson, 2000). At the same time, clinical laboratory tests are an essential component of modern health care and drive other costly diagnostic and therapeutic decisions. As a result of continuing scientific advances, laboratory tests are likely to play an even greater role in the detection, treatment, and monitoring of disease in the twenty-first century.

The incentive of manufacturers to develop new laboratory technologies,[1] and the ability of Medicare beneficiaries to have access to them, are affected by Medicare's payment policy. Medicare's current system of payment for laboratory services in outpatient settings was designed in the early 1980s. Although specific payment rates have changed over the past 20 years, the basic payment methodology has remained unchanged since the early 1980s. The introduction of new technologies and changes in regulations and the laboratory marketplace have had a significant impact on the structure of the laboratory industry during the past 20 years.[2] In the face of these changes, current Medicare payment policy for outpatient clinical laboratory services seems not only outdated, but also irrational. Unless it is changed, the current payment system could eventually inhibit

---

[1]New technology may mean completely new testing techniques; however, it also refers to incremental improvements in testing equipment and reagents.

[2]For the purpose of this report, the clinical laboratory industry refers to laboratories that process and produce laboratory results. When manufacturers of laboratory tests, equipment, and chemicals are included, this will be specified.

innovation and reduce beneficiary access to care (Lewin Group, 2000). Inadequate payment rates could slow the industry's ability to develop and disseminate new technology and laboratories' willingness to adopt valuable but more expensive technologies. The committee did not find a lack of interest in or adoption of innovation, however.

Medicare payment policy influences the laboratory industry's financial health. Medicare payments for outpatient clinical laboratory services represent about 10 percent of the business of clinical laboratories.[3] In part because of repeated cuts in Medicare's payment rates for laboratory tests, the actual amount in real dollars that Medicare spends on outpatient clinical laboratory services has declined.[4] In addition, limited evidence[5] suggests that Medicare payment policy for outpatient clinical laboratory services influences payment policy for some private payers, and Medicare limits are a cap on state Medicaid laboratory payment rates.

Recognizing that Medicare's payment system for clinical laboratory services may have to be modernized, Congress mandated that the Secretary of the Department of Health and Human Services (DHHS) arrange for the Institute of Medicine (IOM) of the National Academies to review the current Medicare payment methodology for outpatient clinical laboratory services and make recommendations to improve the system (Balanced Budget Act of 1997 [BBA], Public Law 105-33). The IOM was selected because it has a unique advisory process in which independent, volunteer experts analyze issues and make policy recommendations.

STATEMENT OF TASK

The Health Care Financing Administration (HCFA), the division of DHHS that administers the Medicare program, interpreted the mandate of Congress and contracted with the IOM to conduct a study to undertake the following:

- Describe the clinical laboratory industry and, where applicable, document significant differences between the situation of this industry today and in the early 1980s, when the current design of Medicare's clinical laboratory payment

---

[3]According to Health Care Financing Administration testimony before the committee and the Office of the Actuary, $3.6 billion was spent on Medicare outpatient clinical laboratory services in 1998. Estimates are that clinical laboratory services are a $35 billion a year industry. See Chapter 2 for more details.

[4]These payment cuts are described in Chapter 4 and were initiated, in part, in response to General Accounting Office (GAO) and Office of the Inspector General (OIG) reports that Medicare was paying too much for laboratory services. See GAO, 1987, 1991. See also OIG reports that found laboratories were inappropriately unbundling test panels and billing Medicare more than physician clients (OIG, 1990, 1996).

[5]CHPS Consulting's (Center for Health Policy Studies) survey of private payers found that six out of nine private health plans base their laboratory payment rates on the Medicare laboratory fee schedule.

methodology was introduced. Factors such as the following should be addressed: the nature and volume of tests performed, sites of testing, the role of automated equipment, reimbursement by public and private payers, access by beneficiaries to services, and quality of testing.

- Document recent trends in laboratory technology and discuss expectations for future trends. Discuss the realized and possible future impacts of these trends on costs, access, and quality of clinical laboratory tests and services.
- Assess the strengths and weaknesses of the current Medicare payment methodology for outpatient laboratory tests. This assessment should include consideration of the role and effectiveness of this methodology in helping to ensure beneficiary access to needed services of high quality, containing costs, and responding to technological changes (both in facilitating access to improved services and in securing the advantages of cost-saving changes in methods of testing).
- Investigate and, if possible, secure and analyze information about costs of performing laboratory tests and about payments made by payers other than Medicare. If possible, present information to help evaluate the effects of laboratory size, specialty, site of service, and geographic location. Tests of particular interest include Pap smears, prostate cancer assays, HIV viral load testing, cancer markers, complete blood counts, and molecular diagnostic testing.
- Describe and assess alternative Medicare payment methodologies. For each option, (1) describe and provide an example of the method; (2) describe in general terms the legislative changes and administrative steps that would be necessary to implement the method; (3) consider the paperwork and financial costs of introducing and using the method for Medicare, the laboratory industry, and physicians and others prescribing tests; and (4) analyze the advantages and disadvantages of the method in comparison to others.

THE IOM STUDY PROCESS

To meet this charge, the IOM put together a 12-member panel of experts composed of laboratorians, physicians, economists, and health care policy and management experts. The committee met five times between January and August 2000 to gather information, deliberate its findings, and formulate recommendations. Background information on the laboratory industry and payment policy was gathered through the use of contractors, literature reviews, testimony, and interviews with key stakeholders and government officials.

The committee found limited data upon which to base its recommendations. For instance, there was limited information on the financial status of different segments of the clinical laboratory industry. Analyses of market share by site of service for Medicare Part B services reported in different publications all cited HCFA data, but reported conflicting findings (Klipp, 2000; Steiner and Root, 1999). There was also very limited information on the cost of performing specific tests and how current Medicare payment amounts compare to test costs and to payments by other purchasers.

To fill this gap, the IOM contracted with CHPS Consulting (Center for Health Policy Studies) of Columbia, Maryland, to conduct a survey of selected health plans to determine their payment rates for 21 laboratory tests plus venipuncture (Appendix C).[6] CHPS Consulting also conducted a limited number of site visits to a variety of laboratory providers to determine their costs of providing a subset of these same laboratory tests. The committee had hoped to get a "snapshot" of costs and payments for these laboratory services from selected sites; however, CHPS Consulting was unable to collect cost data.[7]

The committee also tried to obtain information and input from all relevant stakeholders. All of the information-gathering meetings, as well as presentations made by contractors, were open to the public; attendees were given the opportunity to address the committee at the conclusion of each public meeting; and the committee sought written testimony. Deliberations about recommendations and the report itself were conducted in private, as required by the National Academies' procedures. The closed deliberation process enables committee members to discuss issues independently, without external pressures. IOM senior staff and a panel of external expert reviewers evaluated the report to ensure that the committee met its charge and based its findings and recommendations on sufficient evidence.

During the committee's fact finding, stakeholders identified many different problems related to laboratory coverage, coding, and payment policy that they wanted the committee to address. As the remainder of this report shows, policies in these areas are complex and interrelated. At the same time, however, the committee's charge was narrowly defined. Neither the scope nor the time frame of the contract permitted the committee to go into problems of coverage and coding in depth, but these matters were examined where they touch on payment concerns. The committee believes that many of the problems and issues raised in public testimony transcend the current payment methodology.

GOALS FOR A PAYMENT SYSTEM

During its deliberations, the committee recognized that any payment system ought to be directed toward the achievement of certain goals. The committee agreed on the following five goals for a Medicare payment system for laboratory tests. The way these goals are balanced while crafting policy elements should

---

[6]These tests were selected because they were suggested by the statement of task or because they are at the top of the list in terms of Medicare expenditures for laboratory services and are representative of different types of laboratory tests, such as chemistry, microbiology, and pathology.

[7]The scope of the study was limited by the committee's time frame and budget and by the federal Paperwork Reduction Act, which requires Office of Management and Budget review of federally sponsored surveys of 10 or more respondents.

lead to a payment system that includes incentives for providers and beneficiaries to act as intended—whether to control costs or to utilize needed care. The five goals represent the ideal. Tensions between different goals, however, may make it impossible for all of the goals to be achieved through payment policy alone.[8]

The five goals provide a framework for assessing the strengths and weaknesses of both current and alternative Medicare payment methodologies for clinical laboratory services. In Chapter 6, the options for payment policy are measured against these goals.

1. **Beneficiary access:** Medicare beneficiaries should have access to appropriate services on a timely basis. In the context of clinical laboratory services, three aspects of access are pertinent: medically necessary laboratory tests[9] should be *available* to all Medicare beneficiaries;[10] overly burdensome financial barriers should not limit beneficiary *access* to appropriate services; and finally, *turnaround time*, or the length of time it takes for the physician to get laboratory test results, should not jeopardize quality of care.

2. **Flexibility:** The payment methodology should have formal mechanisms to promptly recognize and determine a fair payment for new technology and to adjust fees that, over time, become unreasonable as a result of both scientific and economic changes. The health care environment is changing rapidly. Changes in medical practice, technology, the cost of providing services, and the Medicare budget all affect the provision of health care services. The payment methodology must be flexible enough to incorporate innovation by efficiently recognizing and paying for cost-effective new technology. In practice, this requires the coding system to respond to new technologies efficiently. There must also be practical data-driven mechanisms to change fees that are inappropriate and to update payment amounts in a timely fashion.

To incorporate innovation and ensure that beneficiaries have access to appropriate care, payment amounts for new technology should be set quickly and then reviewed periodically to ensure that they are reasonable. Neither the payment amount nor the payment policies should adversely affect the appropriate use of new tests, testing methods, or equipment. Because significantly inappropriate fees can create perverse incentives to misuse health care resources along with barriers to beneficiary access, the payment methodology should have a

---

[8]As an example of other goals for payment policy, see the Physician Payment Review Commission (PPRC, 1987).

[9]By law, Medicare only covers services that are "medically necessary." Medical necessity is determined by national and local Medicare coverage policy. These coverage determinations are made based on available outcomes data, local practice patterns, and the consensus of expert panels. References to medical necessity relate to this Medicare definition. Stating that a test is medically necessary does not imply there are substantial outcomes data to support its use, only that Medicare has agreed to cover the test.

[10]Beneficiaries needing laboratory tests often must travel to their physician, the laboratory, or specimen collection site to have the specimen drawn. Payment policy should not exacerbate this burden on beneficiaries.

process, which is open to stakeholder participation, to challenge and change these fees.

A payment system will quickly become outdated unless it incorporates a mechanism to update payment amounts periodically in response to changes in the health care environment. These updates should consider inflation, shifts in the composition of the Medicare population, changes in laboratory technology, and the Medicare budget.

3. **Transparency:** The process for setting payment amounts and payment policies should be understandable and open to input from the public and providers. Increased visibility can diminish the potential for government regulatory agencies over time to become "captured" by the industries they regulate.[11] Generally, if all stakeholders understand the rules of the payment system, understand the rationale behind the rules, and feel they have had an opportunity to influence rule development, they will be more likely to comply with them. It is essential that payment policy be communicated clearly to stakeholders during its formation and following its establishment.

4. **Value:** The payment methodology should promote the purchase of the best-value health care services for beneficiaries. "Best value" is not necessarily "lowest price"; rather, it reflects *efficient* and *appropriate use* of laboratory services with the ultimate goal of producing a positive health outcome for the beneficiary using high-quality, appropriate, health care services. Economic incentives should not drive clinical decisionmaking, and prices should be related to the costs of providing services. Therefore, the payment methodology should encourage clinically appropriate care through the absence of financial incentives to provide a particular type of test or financial barriers that inhibit providing other tests. In addition to establishing value on a test-by-test basis, the payment methodology should promote value in aggregate spending. Thus, the system should promote quality health care generally and should minimize opportunities for waste, fraud, and abuse.

5. **Administrative simplicity and efficiency:** The payment system should strive for simplicity and efficiency in its administrative operations for the provider, payer, and patient. The system should not be unduly burdensome to beneficiaries, physicians, or laboratories. It is important to eliminate any nonessential paperwork and to avoid a design that attempts to accommodate every exceptional case.

To provide context for the remainder of this report, the next two sections of this chapter describe the types of clinical laboratory services covered by the Medicare Part B outpatient fee schedule and outline the basic structure of the Medicare payment system.

---

[11] Some political and economic analysts point out the risk of a government agency, instead of representing the interests of the general public, to unduly take the interests of the firms it regulates into account. This can result in higher costs and may inhibit innovation.

CLINICAL LABORATORY SERVICES COVERED BY MEDICARE

Unless otherwise stated, for the purpose of this report, clinical laboratory services refer to in vitro tests on specimens derived from humans for the purpose of providing information for the diagnosis, prevention, and treatment of disease or impairment or the assessment of health (see Box 1.1). Clinical laboratory services include not only the technical production of tests, but also clinical and analytical advice to the ordering physician from clinical pathologists, chemists, and microbiologists, as needed. Although there are many types of clinical laboratory services, many are not covered by health insurance. Other uses of clinical laboratory services that are not covered by Medicare include screening for drugs

BOX 1.1 Clinical Laboratory Services

Diagnosis

Clinical laboratory tests are often used to help make a diagnosis. Diagnostic tests may look for the presence of an infectious organism, such as a virus or parasite; may find pathology such as cancerous cells; or may help distinguish between different possible causes of a symptom. Examples of diagnostic tests include tests to identify streptococcus bacteria and blood tests that can identify anemia through a low red blood cell count.

Screening

Tests are used for screening purposes when they are performed in the absence of signs, symptoms, complaints, or personal history of disease or injury. Screening tests may provide the opportunity for early intervention that can prevent the onset or spread of disease. Screening tests can also be used as a reference point, establishing a baseline measure that can be helpful in diagnosis in the future. Tests for HIV, Pap smears, prostate-specific antigen, cholesterol level, and specific DNA markers such as BRCA1, which may indicate that the patient has an increased risk for breast cancer, can be used for either screening or diagnosis.

Patient Monitoring

Monitoring tests are used to track disease progression or improvement, identify side effects and complications, monitor drug levels, and assess prognosis. Examples of monitoring tests include blood glucose monitoring for diabetics, tests that measure the levels of seizure medication to ensure that the patient is not being under- or overdosed, and blood T-cell counts that give an indication of the status of HIV infection.

of abuse, conducting forensic investigation, evaluating a person's health for life insurance, and testing as a part of clinical research and drug development. Because they are not covered by the Medicare program, these additional uses of laboratory services are not discussed in detail in this report.

THE MEDICARE PROGRAM

The committee was asked to analyze payment policy for a very specific portion of the Medicare program—clinical laboratory services paid for under the Part B outpatient Medicare benefit. It is important, therefore, to understand the structure of the Medicare program in order to focus on the portion of Medicare payment policy that the committee was asked to evaluate. Title XVIII of the Social Security Act (SSA) created Medicare, an entitlement program that currently provides health care coverage to 38.8 million elderly, or permanently disabled individuals and to people with end-stage renal disease (HCFA, 1999). The Medicare program was designed to make health care accessible to covered beneficiaries and to protect beneficiaries from the financial impact of catastrophic disease and injury. Medicare covers health services that are medically necessary to diagnose and treat disease and injury. Unless specifically authorized by statute, Medicare does not pay for screening tests or preventive care. Coverage for exceptions, such as Pap smears and screening for prostate-specific antigen (PSA), is limited to only one test during a prescribed period of time.

The scope of this study does not include laboratory services ordered for Medicare beneficiaries who have chosen to enroll in a managed care plan or beneficiaries covered by traditional fee-for-service Medicare who are inpatients in hospitals, hospice, or skilled nursing facilities. The managed care and inpatient fee-for-service market segments are reviewed briefly below to distinguish them from the outpatient, fee-for-service market segment.

Although the majority of Medicare beneficiaries rely on traditional Medicare fee-for-service benefits,[12] approximately 16 percent of Medicare beneficiaries currently participate in a Medicare+Choice option, which is typically a managed care plan. Managed care plans are paid a capitated amount for each beneficiary and manage the way they pay providers differently than traditional fee-for-service Medicare. Laboratory services paid through managed care plans are not affected by Medicare Part B payment policy (MCOL, 2000). While the managed care segment of the Medicare market grew during the 1990s, many health plans have recently chosen to discontinue their Medicare managed care plans (Morgan, 2000).

Laboratory tests provided to beneficiaries in traditional fee-for-service Medicare during the course of an inpatient stay, or in the hospital outpatient setting within 72 hours surrounding an inpatient stay, also are excluded from the

---

[12]Fee-for-service means that the provider is paid for every service or bundle of services that is provided.

scope of this study. Medicare pays hospitals a lump sum for an inpatient stay based on the patient's diagnosis. All laboratory services provided as part of an inpatient stay are included in that bundled payment.

This report focuses on the clinical laboratory services ordered by a physician that are covered by Medicare Part B benefits. Participation in Part B coverage, which pays for physician office visits and other outpatient care, is voluntary for Medicare beneficiaries. Because the Part B premium is subsidized through general revenues and is affordable by most beneficiaries, approximately 95 percent of Medicare beneficiaries have Part B coverage.[13]

Approximately 23 insurance carriers and 30 fiscal intermediaries (FIs) process laboratory claims paid under Medicare Part B. The carriers and FIs are contractors to HCFA who provide services in 56 geographic areas across the country.[14] To make claims submission easier for hospital and other facility laboratories, the same FIs that process inpatient claims process all laboratory claims from hospital outpatient departments and other facility laboratories. Carriers process claims from physician offices and independent laboratories.

The methods used to pay for health care services provided under Part B vary. Physicians and laboratories are currently paid based on fee schedules. The list of payment amounts for all clinical laboratory tests in each of the 56 Medicare carrier jurisdictions is called the laboratory fee schedule. The fee schedule has prices for approximately 1,100 separate tests, which pays for the technical component of the test.[15] The current payment methodology was established in 1984 and revised in 1986, but current fees are based on what laboratories were charging for tests in their local area in 1983, adjusted over time. A national cap, called the National Limitation Amount (NLA), limits the amount paid per test.[16] It is this payment methodology for Part B clinical laboratory services, which includes 56 fee schedules limited by the NLA, that the IOM committee was asked to evaluate.

What Types of Laboratory Services Are Included in the Medicare Laboratory Fee Schedule?

Not all tests are included in the Medicare laboratory fee schedule. Medicare requires providers to use numeric codes from the HCFA Common Procedural Coding System (HCPCS) to bill for laboratory services. These codes are used to

---

[13]Out of 38.8 million Medicare beneficiaries, 36.7 million (or 95 percent) participated in Part B in 1998 (HCFA, 1999).

[14]Each carrier region or jurisdiction is roughly equivalent to a state, with some larger states divided into smaller regions.

[15]The PPRC (1995) defines "technical component" as the part of a relative value or fee for a diagnostic test or therapeutic procedure that represents the cost of performing the service excluding the physician's work.

[16]This national cap for each test is currently set at 74 percent of the median of each fee.

describe the laboratory test or test methodology. The HCPCS coding system includes Current Procedural Terminology (CPT) codes assigned and published by the American Medical Association (AMA), plus temporary codes assigned by HCFA or its contractors.[17] The laboratory fee schedule includes CPT codes for medical services in the range of 80000 to 89999 and some additional HCPCS codes. Some of these temporary HCPCS codes have become permanent, such as those for venipuncture and specimen collection. Some laboratory professional services, such as surgical pathology and diagnostic radiology have CPT codes in the 80000–89999 range, but they are paid for under the Medicare fee schedule for physician services[18] and are not part of the clinical laboratory fee schedule.

In addition to these physician services, the following laboratory services are also excluded from the fee schedule:

- laboratory services included in the end stage renal disease (ESRD) program package ofservices;
- laboratory services provided to patients in a skilled nursing facility;
- tests related to blood banking or blood products;
- physiological testing, imaging, and electrocardiograms (EKGs); and
- dental laboratory services.

ORGANIZATION OF THE REPORT

Both the legislative mandate and the charge from HCFA to the IOM for preparation of this report reflect the importance of putting Medicare payment policy in the broader context of payment for services provided by the laboratory industry as a whole, reviewing and analyzing trends in the health care environment, and anticipating developments in laboratory technology. This report is organized along the lines of specific elements of the charge to the IOM.

The next three chapters provide background information on clinical laboratories and Medicare payment policy. Chapter 2 reviews the clinical laboratory industry as a whole; its Medicare outpatient market segment; and the way environmental trends in regulation, government efforts to reduce waste and abuse, and payment levels have affected the industry. It concludes with a discussion of how the industry has responded to these trends. Chapter 3 discusses anticipated trends in automation, information technology, and laboratory testing technology, as well as expected shifts in site of service and laboratory staffing needs. Chapter 4 describes the current Medicare payment system and how it has evolved. The vari-

---

[17]For instance, HCFA assigned HCPCS codes for Pap smears conducted for screening purposes to facilitate billing for this newly approved use of the test. HCPCS temporary codes often can be assigned more quickly than CPT codes which facilitates the billing of new technology.

[18]The "professional component" is defined as the part of a relative value or fee that represents the cost of a physician's interpretation of a diagnostic test or treatment planning for a therapeutic procedure (PPRC, 1995).

ous elements of a payment methodology are described and form the framework for analyzing the current outpatient clinical laboratory payment system.

The last three chapters present the committee's conclusions about the current payment system and possible alternatives. Chapter 5 assesses the current system in light of the payment policy goals that the committee has articulated in this chapter. Chapter 6 examines alternative payment methods that could be used by Medicare. Chapter 7 presents the committee's recommendations, based on its assessment of the current system and the benefits and feasibility of several modifications to it.

REFERENCES

Gustafson, T. January 20, 2000. Testimony before the IOM Committee on Medicare Payment Methodology for Clinical Laboratory Services. Washington, DC.

General Accounting Office (GAO). December 1987. Medicare: Lab Fee Schedules Produce Large Beneficiary Savings but No Program Savings. HRD-88-32. Washington, DC: GAO.

GAO. June 1991. Medicare Payments for Clinical Laboratory Test Services are too High. HRD-91-59. Washington, DC: GAO.

Health Care Financing Administration (HCFA). 1999. "Medicare Enrollment Trends, 1966–1998." Web page, [accessed 6 July 2000]. Available at www.hcfa.gov/stats/enrltrnd.htm.

Klipp, J. 2000. *Lab Industry Strategic Outlook 2000: Market Trends & Analysis*. Washington, DC: Washington G-2 Reports.

Lewin Group. 2000. *Outlook for Medical Technology Innovation: Will Patients Get the Care They Need? Report 1: The State of the Industry*. Washington, DC: The Health Industry Manufacturers Association.

Managed Care On-Line (MCOL). 2000. Medicare+Choice Enrollment Penetration by State. Webpage: accessed July 6, 2000. Available at http://www.medicarehmo.com/mrepenrp.thm.

Morgan, D. June 30, 2000. More health plans quit Medicare. *Washington Post,* section A, p. 8.

Office of the Inspector General (OIG). January 1990. Changes are Needed in the Way Medicare Pays for Clinical Laboratory Tests. A-09-89-00031. Washington, DC: OIG.

OIG. January 1996. Follow-up Report to "Changes are Needed in the Way Medicare Pays for Clinical Laboratory Tests." A-09-93-00056. Washington, DC: OIG.

Physician Payment Review Commission (PPRC). 1987. *Annual Report to Congress, 1987*. Washington, DC: PPRC.

PPRC. 1995. *Annual Report to Congress, 1995*. Washington, DC: PPRC.

Steiner, J. W., and J. M. Root. June 1999. The battle between hospital and commercial labs: Who's winning? *Clinical Laboratory News,* p. 4.

2
Background and Environmental Trends

This chapter provides background on the clinical laboratory industry and analyzes trends in the health care environment that have affected the cost of providing clinical laboratory services, the quality of those services, and beneficiary access to care. An understanding of these factors, in addition to an appreciation of anticipated trends in laboratory technology (discussed in greater detail in Chapter 3) is necessary to design a forward-thinking, effective Medicare outpatient clinical laboratory payment system and anticipate its likely effects.[1]

A cautionary note is necessary at the beginning of this chapter. Reliable descriptive data on the clinical laboratory industry are extremely limited, and any picture the committee attempts to paint will be frustratingly hazy.[2] There are a number of factors that influence the quality of available data. First, no single industry association or public agency oversees all aspects of this industry, and there is no unique census Standard Industrial Classification (SIC) business code

---

[1]Much of the research for this chapter draws on work conducted by CHPS Consulting (Center for Health Policy Studies) Columbia, Maryland, for the Institute of Medicine (IOM).

[2]Multiple statistics citing the Health Care Financing Administration (HCFA) as the data source often did not match, perhaps because HCFA produces volumes of data that are continuously updated, making the time and specific definitions of data elements critical to understanding what the data represent. Many HCFA data come from ongoing program operations developed to serve claims processing needs rather than policy research interests; thus, different analysts may manipulate the raw data somewhat differently resulting in numbers that vary slightly.

for clinical laboratory services; therefore, there are no standard data sources or common definitions used for data that are collected. Second, large companies and hospitals often provide other laboratory services in addition to clinical laboratory testing, and these services may be included in aggregate data for laboratory testing.[3] Finally, laboratory services are only a small segment of a hospital's or physician's business and often are not calculated or are reported separately. Where necessary, this chapter cites several data sources when there is no obvious "right" one. The general direction of the trends described in this chapter is more important than the exact values of various figures.

BACKGROUND ON THE CLINICAL LABORATORY INDUSTRY

The clinical laboratory industry is very diverse. Understanding the different types of laboratories, their markets, and the types of services they provide is critical because each has an effect on the cost and quality of laboratory services, as well as beneficiary access to care. This section discusses the number, types, and geographic distribution of laboratories; testing volume; revenue distribution by type of laboratory; and an analysis of the trends in spending for laboratory services in relation to other health care services. It concludes with an analysis of the financial strength of the industry.

Sites of Service

In 1999, 170,102 laboratories conducted 5.7 billion laboratory tests for both inpatients and outpatients in the United States (Tables 2.1 and 2.2). There are three main types of laboratories that provide clinical laboratory services: hospital-based, independent, and physician office laboratories (POLs).

- **Hospital-based laboratories:** Hospital-based laboratories conduct more tests than all other types of laboratories combined. They serve primarily the inpatient and outpatient testing needs of their hospital but may also conduct tests for patients not seen at their hospital, typically called "outreach testing." In 1999, 8,560 hospital-based laboratories (Table 2.1) conducted almost 3 billion laboratory tests (Table 2.2). There are many more hospital-based laboratories than there are hospitals in the U.S. because some hospitals operate more than one laboratory. Independent laboratories run some hospital-based laboratories.
- **Independent laboratories:** Independent laboratories conduct tests for physicians, hospitals, and other health care providers. These laboratories tend to be regional in nature, with single companies operating multiple laboratory fa-

[3]For example, data on revenue may include revenue from testing related to life insurance and testing for drugs of abuse.

TABLE 2.1 Number of Laboratories by Type of Facility; 1999–Early 2000

Type of Facility	Number of Laboratories	Percentage of Total
Hospital laboratories	8,560	5
Independent laboratories	4,936	3
Physician office laboratories	105,089	62
Other	51,517	30
Total	170,102	

SOURCE: Health Care Financing Administration, 2000a.

TABLE 2.2 Test Volume by Type of Facility; 1999–Early 2000

Type of Facility	Volume (millions)	Percentage of Total
Hospital laboratories	2,958.2	52
Independent laboratories	1,514.2	26
Physician office laboratories	656.4	11
Other	597.1	10
Total	5,725.9	

NOTE: Volume figures include both inpatient and outpatient tests performed for all public and private sector payers.

SOURCE: Health Care Financing Administration, 2000a.

cilities. In 1999, 4,936 independent laboratories (Table 2.1) conducted almost 1.5 billion laboratory tests in the United States (26 percent) (Table 2.2). The number of independent laboratories is somewhat misleading because independent laboratories underwent rapid corporate consolidation during the 1990s, resulting in two large national and many other smaller independent laboratories.[4] Multiple laboratories that may be counted separately are actually part of one corporate entity.

• **Physician office laboratories:** POLs generally conduct relatively simple or moderately complex tests to provide immediate, on-site results to physicians. At 105,089, there are far more POLs than other types of laboratories (Table 2.1). While many POLs conduct only the most simple laboratory tests and have very

[4]Quest Diagnostics Inc. recently took over SmithKline Beecham's clinical laboratory business to form the largest independent laboratory. Its closest competitor is LabCorp.

low test volume, others may serve large group practices and provide a range of tests at volumes comparable to those of independent laboratories.

• **Other laboratories:** The remaining laboratories include testing facilities at end-stage renal disease (ESRD) centers, home health agencies, nursing homes, and other sites. Although these "other laboratories" account for slightly more than 30 percent of all laboratory facilities (Table 2.1), they conduct only 10 percent of all laboratory tests (Table 2.2) and are often not paid out of the Medicare outpatient laboratory benefit. Trends in numbers of laboratories and testing volume broken down by more specific type of service provider are presented in Appendix D.

Since some types of tests are complex or require special expertise, they may be sent from one laboratory to another. Laboratories that conduct tests for other laboratories are called "reference" laboratories. Reference laboratories are usually large and may be independent or hospital based. Some tests are so uncommon, complex, expensive, and dependent on specialized interpretation skill that they are labeled "esoteric." Some tests previously considered esoteric, such as polymerase chain reaction (PCR) testing for HIV, have become so common that the esoteric label no longer applies. Laboratories that specialize in esoteric testing are usually affiliated with a university or research institution but may be independent.

Geographic Distribution

Clinical laboratories in the United States are geographically distributed much like the population. According to a 1995 summary report of the Clinical Laboratory Improvement Advisory Committee of the Centers for Disease Control and Prevention (CDC), Texas and California have the greatest number of laboratories, while Midwestern and rural New England states have the lowest concentration (CDC, 1995).

Size and Distribution of the Market

The clinical laboratory industry is a $30 billion to $35 billion industry [5] (Dyckman and Cassidy, 2000; Klipp, 2000; Merrill Lynch, 1999) representing approximately 3.5 percent of the $1.0 trillion in total personal health care expenditures in the United States in 1998. Based on recent pricing trends, CHPS Consulting estimates that expenditures on laboratory tests in 1999 are expected to be 3–6 percent higher than for 1998 (Dyckman and Cassidy, 2000). Because hospitals are paid for inpatient care based largely on per-case and per diem payment methodologies, rather than on a fee-for-service (FFS) basis, payments for laboratory services provided in the inpatient setting are included within

[5] This includes both inpatient and outpatient testing services.

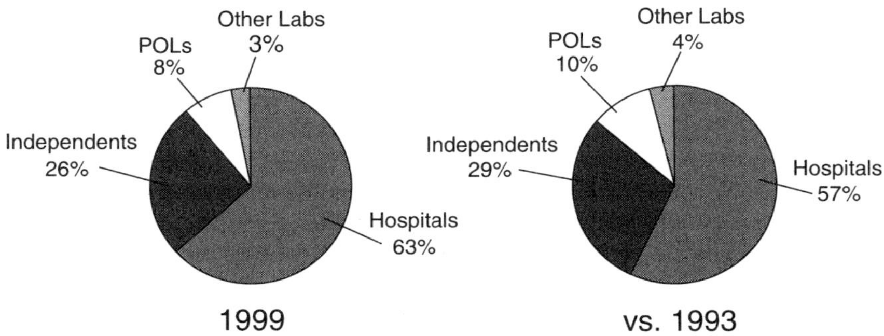

FIGURE 2.1 Laboratory industry revenue by segment, 1999. SOURCE: Klipp (2000).

payments for more broadly defined services. This is explained further in the discussion of environmental trends below.

Not surprisingly, hospital-based laboratories, which have the highest test volume, also have the largest market share in terms of revenue. Industry sources put the hospital-based market share at 63 percent for 1999. This is an increase from the estimated 57 percent share it held in 1993 (Figure 2.1). Independent laboratories hold about 26 percent of the market share, while "other" laboratories account for only 3 percent. Although POLs represent about 11 percent of test volume, they receive only 8 percent of the revenue because they tend to perform simpler, less expensive tests.

Trends in Expenditures for Laboratory Services

The early 1980s was a period of significant health care inflation, and during that time, clinical laboratories benefited from favorable payment policies. Beginning with implementation of the inpatient prospective payment system (PPS) in the mid-1980s, and with the growth of managed care in the late 1980s and 1990s, changes to both governmental and nongovernmental payment systems helped rein in health care spending and bring health care inflation back into the single digits.

Expenditures for laboratory services have been particularly affected by efforts to control health care costs. While the *rate* of growth in national health expenditures has slowed, *actual* expenditures for most categories of health care spending have continued to increase even when controlling for inflation (Figure 2.2). In contrast, expenditures for laboratory services provided in all settings have declined steadily; expenditures in 1998 were more than 10 percent lower than in 1993 (Klipp, 2000). Figure 2.3 tracks the trends in health expenditures for the five years from 1993 to 1998 for total personal health care, laboratory, hospital, and physician services.

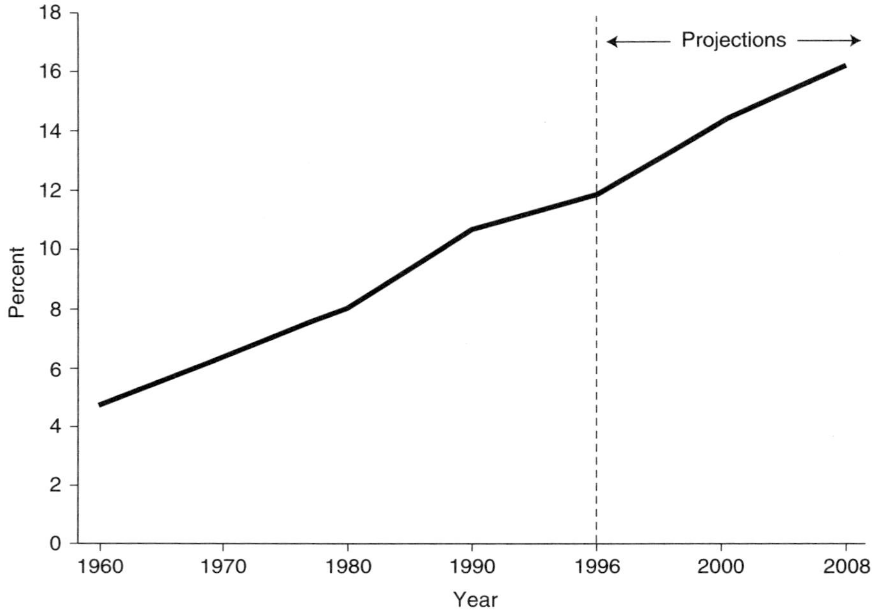

FIGURE 2.2 Personal health care expenditures as a percentage of Gross Domestic Product: 1960–2008. SOURCE: Health Care Financing Administration, data from the Office of Strategic Planning and the Office of National Health Statistics.

Financial Strength of the Laboratory Industry

The committee searched for direct evidence of the financial health of the clinical laboratory industry, but found little because most segments of the industry are not required to report financial information. POLs and outpatient hospital laboratories are not independent businesses, but integrated parts of physicians' practices and hospitals, respectively. Also, many commercial independent laboratories, particularly relatively small laboratories, are not publicly held corporations and have no obligation to report financial data publicly. To assess the financial health of the industry, therefore, the committee reviewed a number of finance industry reports as well as recent market studies that provide some information on the commercial laboratory industry's profitability, mostly for the largest laboratory firms (Donaldson, 1993; Lehman Brothers, 1993; Merrill Lynch, 1999; Smith Barney Research, 1990). The committee supplemented this information with indirect evidence of industry financial health, such as changes in number, volume, and market share of the different segments.

The committee found virtually no direct information on the financial performance of POLs; however, the number of POLs continues to grow, indicating that there is some incentive to provide these services. Because of incentives re-

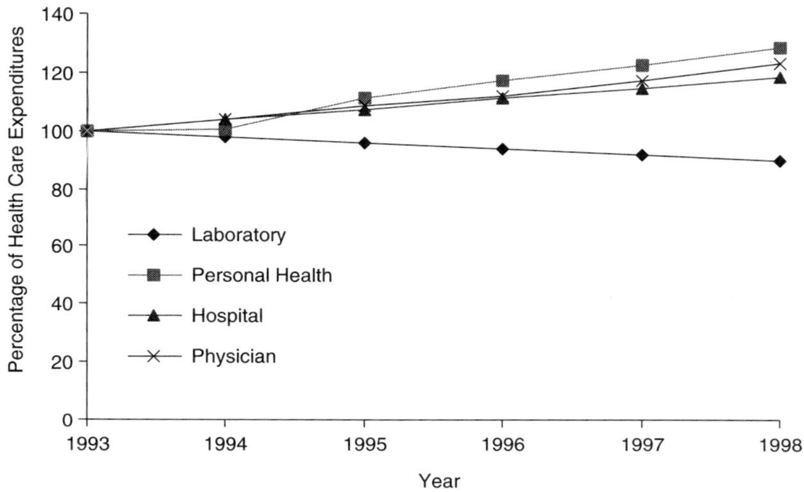

FIGURE 2.3 Trends in expenditures for health care services, 1993–1998. SOURCE: Laboratory data: CHPS Consulting analysis of information in Klipp (2000); other health services: Levit et. al. (2000).

lated to efficiency and convenience, physicians may provide laboratory services regardless of their independent profitability.

The committee also found no direct data to assess the financial well being of hospital-based laboratories. Hospital-based laboratories' share of the total market grew during the 1990s, despite payment reductions and the aggressiveness of managed care contracting. Most, if not all, of this growth has been in the provision of laboratory services in the hospital's *outpatient* department and for providers outside the hospital (outreach testing).

The growth in outreach testing can be attributed to diametrically opposed circumstances. Growth may suggest that, as a group, hospital-based laboratories are profitable. On the other hand, it could be a response to market changes that threaten the financial viability of hospitals, including global shifts from inpatient to outpatient care. In this case, growth may reflect an attempt by hospitals to spread fixed costs across an increased volume of services.

Available data do not reflect the experience of hospital laboratories after implementation of the Balanced Budget Act of 1997 (BBA), which changed inpatient payment and mandated a new payment methodology for outpatient services. The new prospective payment system for outpatient hospital services does not include laboratory services, but could affect the general financial status of hospitals. Changes mandated by the 1999 Balanced Budget Refinement Act (BBRA) for the new outpatient PPS is expected to lessen the negative projected financial effect on hospitals (Guterman, 2000).

Environmental factors during the 1990s, particularly reductions in Medicare fees and growth in managed care among both public and private payers, had a significant effect on the profitability of the independent laboratory sector (Hoerger et al., 1996). By 1995, all of the laboratory industry's leading firms were either experiencing losses or sharply declining profits. According to Klipp (2000), in 1996, the top three independent laboratories had a combined net loss of $792 million on $4.58 billion of revenue.

Industry reports suggest that independent laboratories are again becoming profitable. Profit margins improved during the past two years, at least among the major laboratory firms, partly as a result of improved pricing for managed care business. The three largest laboratory firms were marginally profitable in 1998, with an average profit margin of 2.6 percent. In the first half of 1999, after Quest Diagnostics acquired SmithKline Beecham laboratories, the average profit margin for the two largest laboratories, Quest Diagnostics and LabCorp, was 1.2 percent (Klipp, 2000). Stock values for both increased substantially in the first half of 2000. Analysts predict that these companies will be able to streamline production and negotiate better rates for supplies. The committee found no direct financial information on the smaller independent laboratories, which mostly compete in local markets.

MEDICARE PART B CLINICAL LABORATORY TRENDS

Medicare is the largest single purchaser of clinical laboratory services. This section describes Medicare as a segment of the outpatient clinical laboratory market.

Medicare Part B Spending

Laboratory services paid for under the Medicare Part B clinical laboratory fee schedule represent a relatively small component of the annual Medicare budget—about 1.6 percent; however, they constitute a significant portion of the market for the laboratory industry, and Medicare's policies appear to influence the behavior of other payers. According to industry estimates, Medicare pays approximately 29 percent of the nation's laboratory bill when inpatient testing, FFS outpatient testing, and managed care are included (Figure 2.4). The Medicare Part B fee schedule for outpatient laboratory services accounts for approximately one-third of what Medicare spends for laboratory services (Gustafson, 2000).

The Health Care Financing Administration (HCFA) reports that Medicare Part B spending for clinical laboratory services fell from $3.8 billion in 1992 to

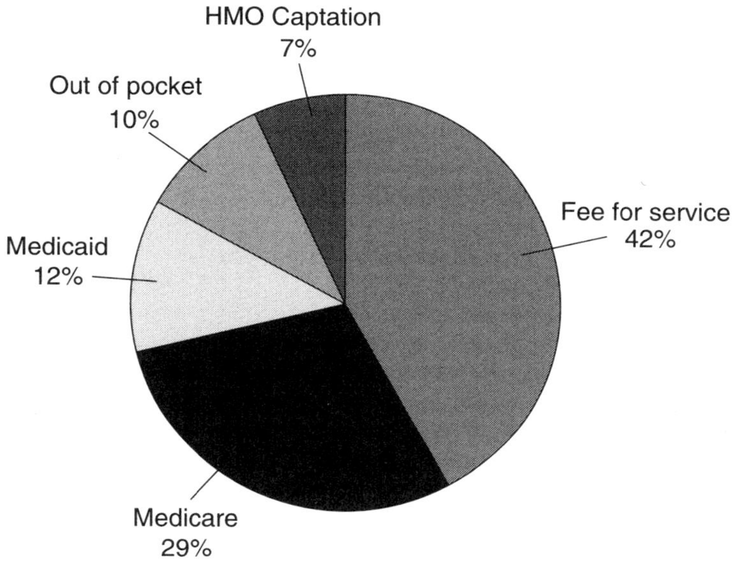

FIGURE 2.4 Laboratory industry payer mix by percentage of revenue, 1999.

$3.6 billion in 1998, with a compound annual growth rate of –1.1 percent (Table 2.3) (Gustafson, 2000). Over the same period, total annual Medicare spending grew from $141 billion to $231 billion; a compound annual growth rate of 8.5 percent (Gustafson, 2000). Clinical laboratory spending as a percentage of total Medicare spending over time is presented in Figure 2.5. Payments for laboratory services per Medicare beneficiary in the FFS program declined during the mid 1990s, but, based on projections, have recently begun to rise (Table 2.4). The Office of the Actuary at HCFA projects that recent growth will continue.

Estimates provided by HCFA show that in 1998, Medicare paid facilities (outpatient-hospital laboratories plus ESRD clinics, nursing homes, home health, and other laboratories) $1,489 million, independent laboratories $1,336 million, and POLs $752 million (Figure 2.6).[6]

---

[6]Medicare does not collect data on its laboratory expenditures by site of service; instead, annual expenditure data are collected based on whether the claim was processed by a Medicare carrier (which processes claims from POLs and independent laboratories) or by a fiscal intermediary (which processes all hospital claims and most other laboratory claims). Any data describing Medicare Part B market share for POLs versus independent laboratories are estimated by subtracting claims that have a physician provider number on them.

TABLE 2.3 Part B Clinical Laboratory Spending by Type of Laboratory

Type of Laboratory	Calendar Year ($ millions)			CAGR, 1992–1998 (%)
	1992	1995	1998	
Independent	1,761	1,871	1,336	–4.5
POL	1,101	936	752	–6.2
Facility [a]	967	1,378	1,489	+7.5
Total	3,829	4,185	3,577	–1.1

NOTE: CAGR = compound annual growth rate.

[a] Includes Part B payments to hospitals, nursing homes, home health agencies, and other laboratories paid by fiscal intermediaries.

SOURCE: Gustafson, 2000.

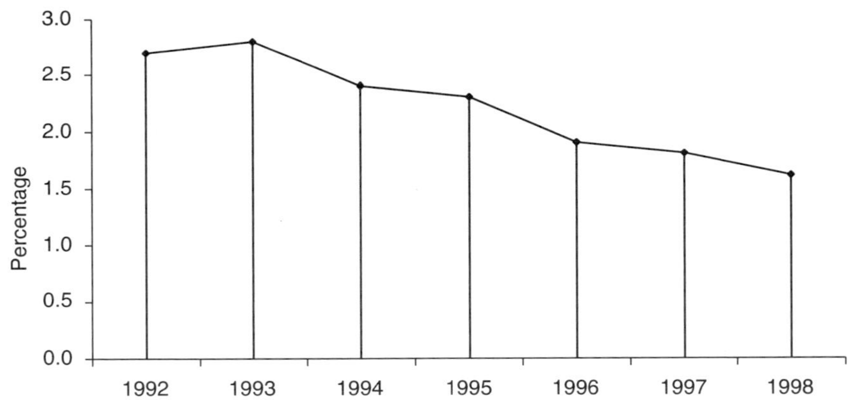

FIGURE 2.5 Part B spending on clinical laboratory services as a percentage of total Medicare spending, 1992–1998. NOTE: Percentages are for total Part B spending on clinical laboratory services, including hospital outpatient/outreach services. SOURCE: Health Care Financing Administration.

Trend data show that the Medicare Part B market share for facilities is growing (Figure 2.7).[7] HCFA's Office of the Actuary projects that this trend will continue. It projects that by 2001, 45 percent of expenditures for services on the clinical laboratory fee schedule will go to the facilities described above, and 55

[7]There is some variation in trend data that may be the result of how various sites of service are defined and whether "other laboratories" are included within the outpatient hospital segment.

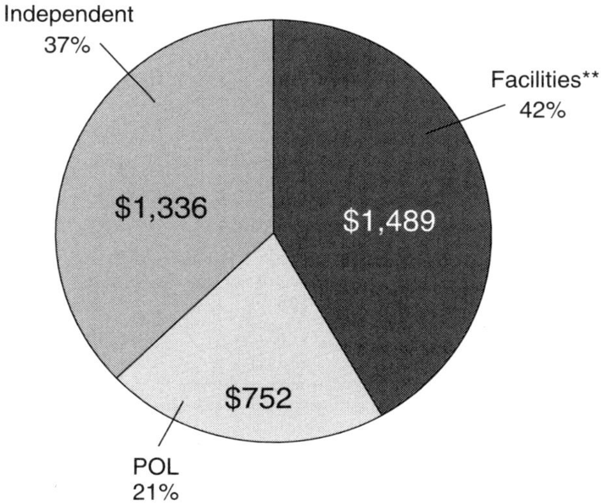

FIGURE 2.6 Medicare Part B spending (in millions)* by laboratory type, 1998. Includes carrier and FI data for the laboratory fee schedule and some physician services such as pathology. **Includes outpatient hospital, ESRD, nursing homes, home health, and other laboratory services paid for by FIs. SOURCE: Health Care Financing Administration.

percent will go to independent and physician office laboratories (Steiner and Root, 1999).

Although the Medicare Part B fee schedule for clinical laboratory services covers approximately 1,100 different test codes, which reflect an even greater number of tests,[8] the top 10 test codes account for 24 percent and the top 200 account for more than half of Part B laboratory expenditures (Gustafson, 2000).[9]

ENVIRONMENTAL TRENDS

Various environmental trends during the past two decades have put pressure on the clinical laboratory industry to cut costs and improve quality. This section reviews government regulatory efforts to improve quality, protect workers, and reduce waste and abuse. It also reviews cost-control efforts undertaken by both

---

[8]Up from 881 codes in 1994.

[9]The fee schedule for each CPT code for each carrier region and the national limitation amount is available on the Internet at http://www.hcfa.gov/stats/cpt/clfdown.htm.

TABLE 2.4 Part B Laboratory Payments Per FFS Beneficiary, 1995–2002

Year	FFS Enrollment (millions)	Payments per FFS Beneficiary (dollars)		
		Carrier	Intermediary	Total
1995	28.5	177.23	38.72	215.95
1996	27.9	162.21	41.38	203.59
1997	27.1	158.50	44.31	202.81
1998	26.3	160.43	51.09	211.52
1999	25.9	163.45	53.73	217.18
2000	25.1	168.21	56.33	224.54
2001	24.5	174.78	58.86	233.64
2002	24.1	181.76	61.48	243.24

NOTE: FFS = fee-for-service.

SOURCE: Gustafson, 2000.

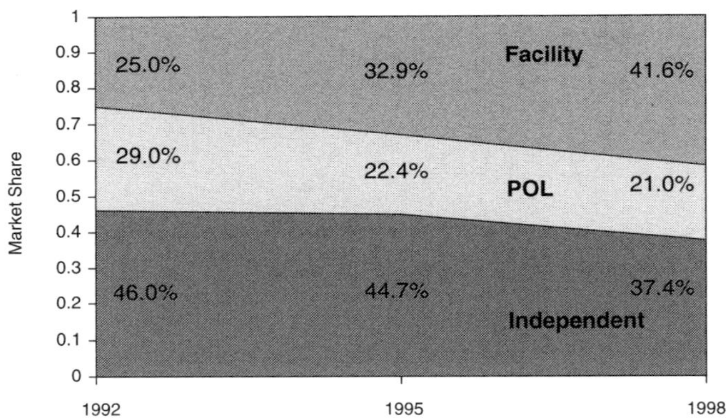

FIGURE 2.7 Medicare Part B market share trends, 1992–1998. SOURCE: T. Gustafson, Health Care Financing Administration, presentation before the IOM committee, January 2000.

public and private payers, particularly new payment policies and aggressive managed care contracting. Although drawing broad conclusions is difficult because the laboratory industry is so diverse, it appears that overall, the quality of clinical laboratory testing has improved and Medicare spending for laboratory services has declined, even while the number of tests per beneficiary has increased. There is no evidence that beneficiary access to care has declined.

Regulatory Trends

Regulatory efforts designed to increase the quality of testing, protect worker safety, and reduce waste and abuse, have increased the cost and administrative burden of providing laboratory services. Data suggest that efforts to improve quality have been successful. Data regarding the effect of regulations to protect workers and reduce waste and abuse are not available.

Clinical Laboratory Improvement Amendments of 1988

Enactment of the Clinical Laboratory Improvement Amendments of 1988 (CLIA) was the most significant factor influencing the general regulatory structure of the laboratory industry in the United States during the past 20 years. In the mid-1980s, a series of *Wall Street Journal* articles exposed major deficiencies in cytology testing (Bogdanich, 1987a; 1987b; see also Inhorn et al., 1994).[10] The medical literature also reported deficiencies in the overall quality of clinical laboratory services (Rej and Jenny, 1992). These articles raised public concern about the quality of the clinical laboratory industry and were a major impetus behind the passage of CLIA. Before the 1988 amendments, the original Clinical Laboratory Improvement Act (1967) regulated laboratories that engaged in interstate commerce, which included most independent laboratories. The 1988 amendments expanded the scope of regulatory authority.

The purpose of CLIA is to "ensure the accuracy, reliability, and timeliness of patient test results regardless of where the test was performed" (HCFA, 1998). The final regulations for CLIA[11] established quality standards and a regulatory structure for all clinical laboratory testing. Under CLIA, a laboratory is defined as any facility that performs laboratory testing on specimens derived from humans for the purpose of providing information for the diagnosis, prevention, assessment, or treatment of disease or impairment of health.

CLIA brought many previously unregulated facilities, particularly POLs, into the regulatory structure. It linked the level of regulatory oversight to the complexity of the testing conducted in the laboratory, rather than focusing on the type of laboratory (physician office, independent, or hospital-based laboratory). This approach helped ensure test site neutrality and established the prem-

---

[10]The *Wall Street Journal* ran a series of newspaper articles that brought national attention to clinical laboratory errors. The articles focused on the high rate of false negative results associated with Pap smear testing. They described a poorly regulated cytology industry, which permitted practices that resulted in perverse incentives for laboratory staff, such as paying on a per-slide basis, providing bonuses for exceeding a total slide-per-day number, and taking slides home for screening. According to the reports, technicians could meet daily quotas at two or more work sites, and some laboratories employed technicians with questionable education and training credentials.

[11]Published in the *Federal Register*, February 28, 1992.

ise that the quality of testing and test results should be the same regardless of where the test is performed (Chapin and Baron, 1995).

Test Complexity and Laboratory Certification

CLIA requires tests to be designated as waived, moderate complexity, or high complexity. The Food and Drug Administration (FDA) has recently taken responsibility for categorizing the level of complexity of new tests.[12] Waived tests are simple to conduct, highly trained staff is not needed, and the chances for error are small. Performance of moderate-complexity and high-complexity tests requires higher levels of expertise. Laboratories performing high-complexity testing must meet stringent personnel requirements.

Since the introduction of CLIA, there has been tremendous growth in the number of waived tests. As of June 2000, the CDC lists almost 750 different waived laboratory testing products for more than 40 types of tests (CDC, 2000). For example, there are 14 different rapid strep test products. For the past few years, waived tests have accounted for approximately 6 percent of all tests conducted, including both inpatient and outpatient testing (HCFA, 2000a). Approximately 40 percent of waived tests are performed in POLs and fewer than 4 percent are performed in independent laboratories.

Table 2.5 presents the most recent available breakdown of test volume for waived and nonwaived tests by type of laboratory. More detailed CLIA test volume data for 1996–2000 are provided in Appendix D.

TABLE 2.5 Waived versus Nonwaived Test Volume, 1999–Early 2000

	Test Volume (millions)			
Type of Facility	Waived Tests[a]	Nonwaived Tests	Total	Waived as a % of Total
Hospital laboratories	95.4	2,862.8	2,958.2	3.2
Independent laboratories	15.1	1,499.1	1,514.2	1.0
Physician office laboratories	160.0	496.4	656.4	24.4
Other	112.5	484.6	597.1	18.8
Total	383.0	5,342.9	5,725.9	6.7

[a] According to the CDC Web site, there are almost 750 testing products that the FDA (previously the CDC) has granted waived status. These tests can be performed in laboratories with minimal regulatory oversight.

SOURCE: Health Care Financing Administration, 2000a.

[12]Prior to 2000, it was the CDC's responsibility.

Since 1996 (the earliest date for which HCFA has CLIA test volume data), the ratio of waived to total tests conducted in the different types of facilities has remained relatively steady (see Figure 2.8).

The extent to which a laboratory can perform different levels of tests depends on its certification.[13] Laboratories that perform tests that are more complex are subject to a higher level of federal regulatory oversight and must adhere to more stringent personnel requirements. Laboratories that wish to perform anything more complex than waived tests or provider-performed microscopy (PPM) are surveyed routinely by either HCFA state inspectors or a private accrediting organization (HCFA, 1998). They also must develop a comprehensive quality assurance and quality control (QA/QC) program.[14]

The CLIA QA/QC program requires laboratories to conduct proficiency (accuracy) testing (PT). PT surveys compare test results for identical samples across clinical laboratories. PT programs aim to identify laboratories with systematic problems that produce errors (as indicated by sustained unacceptable performance), rather than those with an occasional random mistake (Boone, 1992). CLIA requires that clinical laboratories identify the impact of errors by reporting incidents of errors that harmed, or had the potential to harm, the patient.[15]

---

[13]Laboratories receive one of five different certification types:

1. **Certificate of Waiver:** This allows a laboratory to perform only waived tests. Laboratories must register with HCFA and follow the manufacturer's instructions.
2. **Certificate for Provider-Performed Microscopy (PPM) Procedures:** This allows physicians, midlevel practitioners, or dentists to perform PPM procedures and to perform waived tests. A list of PPM procedures can be found at http://www.hcfa.gov/medicaid/clia/ppmplst.htm.
3. **Certificate of Registration:** This allows a laboratory to conduct moderate- or high-complexity laboratory testing or both until the entity is determined by survey to be in compliance with CLIA regulations.
4. **Certificate of Compliance:** This is issued to a laboratory after an inspection that finds the laboratory to be in compliance with all applicable CLIA requirements.
5. **Certificate of Accreditation:** This is issued to a laboratory on the basis of the laboratory's accreditation by an organization approved by HCFA. To receive this certificate, the laboratory must be in compliance with all applicable CLIA requirements.

[14]This QA/QC program must cover evaluations of the effectiveness of clinical laboratory policies and procedures; identification and correction of problems; assurance of accurate, reliable, and timely reporting of test results; and assessments of the adequacy and competency of the staff.

[15]Concern about missing a case of disease has encouraged laboratories to over diagnose (label a result as positive if it is equivocal). Yet, over diagnosis also causes harm by leading to additional testing, anxiety, and even unnecessary treatment.

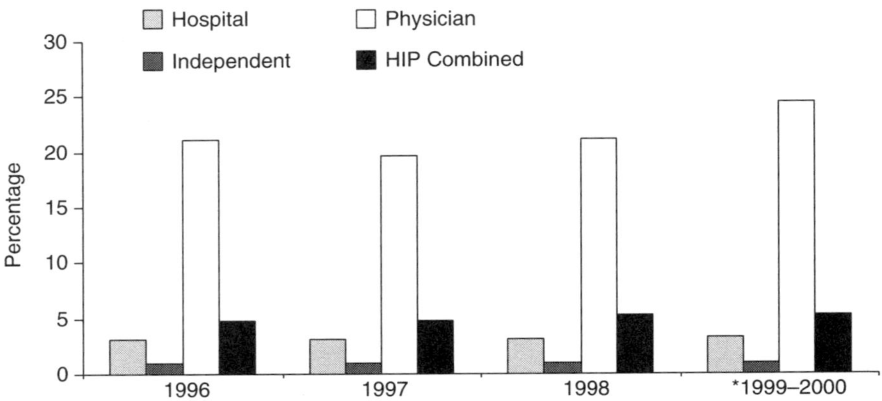

FIGURE 2.8 Waived tests as a percentage of total test volume, 1996–1999, early 2000. SOURCE: Health Care Financing Administration (2000a).

CLIA's Impact on the Laboratory Industry

CLIA increased the regulatory burden for all laboratories. Because CLIA made POLs subject to regulation for the first time, a number of POLs chose to close rather than pay the added cost of licensing fees and QA/QC requirements. Peers & Co. estimated that POL market share (by revenue) decreased from 28 percent in 1986 to 15 percent in 1996 (Hoerger, et al., 1996). Surveys of practitioners both prior to and following CLIA implementation found the following:

- Some physicians, particularly solo practitioners, chose to close their laboratories in response to CLIA.
- Other physicians stopped providing moderate- and high-complexity tests.
- Many physicians believed that CLIA increased the cost and administrative burden of providing laboratory services, but many also believed that CLIA contributed to higher-quality testing (Binns et al., 1998; Born and Thran, 1998; Roussel, 1996; Strauss et al., 1995).

While the cost of implementing CLIA may have been significant for some POLs, other findings suggest that POLs may have closed prematurely. A survey by the Office of the Inspector General (OIG) of a sample of POLs that decided to close found that more than half of the practices in the study reported closing between passage of the amendments in 1988 and their implementation in 1992. The final regulations were actually more liberal than those originally proposed.

As the industry has adjusted to the additional requirements imposed by CLIA, the POL sector has begun to grow again. In 1996, there were 97,542 CLIA-

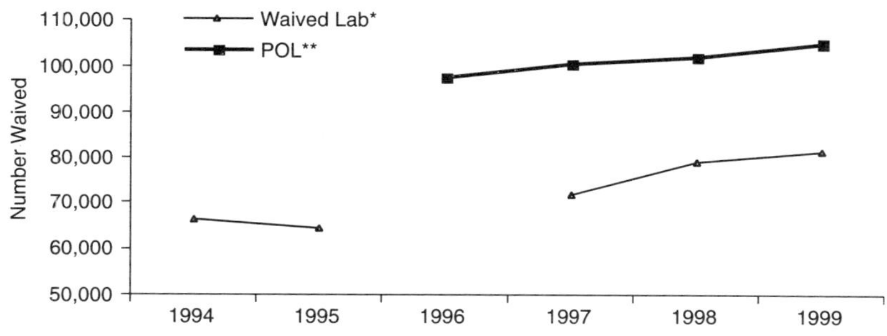

FIGURE 2.9 Comparison of the growth in the number of waived laboratories and POLs, 1994–1999. *SOURCE: Health Care Financing Administration CLIA database (July 1999). Note: Does not include waived laboratories in exempt states, which most years comprised an additional 6,000–7,000 laboratories. Note also that data were unavailable for 1996. **SOURCE: HCFA CLIA database (March 2000). Note: datapoint for 1999 includes 2000 data through March.

registered POLs; by 2000, this number had grown to 105,089 (Figure 2.9 and Appendix D). The volume of testing by POLs also increased (see Appendix D).

There are various explanations for this growth. Some speculate that it is attributable to the dramatic increase in the number of new tests that have achieved waived status.[16] This means that POLs can conduct more tests without facing the regulatory burdens associated with moderate- and high-complexity tests. In addition, the PPM subcategory was added for these types of tests performed by physicians for their own patients. POLs certified to perform PPM may also perform waived tests. Three-quarters of POLs conduct only PPM and waived tests (Figure 2.10). Others think that providers are simply becoming more comfortable with the regulatory environment, and some managed care organizations may be encouraging the use of POLs when it is cost-effective to do so (Auxter, 1999). Still others speculate that the rise may be due in part to pressure from HCFA to register previously unregistered POLs that are attempting to bill Medicare (Auxter, 1999). CLIA increased the cost of providing laboratory services in independent and hospital-based laboratories, but there is no clear evidence that CLIA has created barriers to beneficiary access.[17] Minor declines in the numbers of hospital-based and independent laboratories are likely the result of the con-

---

[16]Klipp (2000), states that the number of waived test products has more than tripled since 1993.

[17]At the time CLIA was enacted, the number of POLs providing moderate-complexity testing declined, and this may have increased turnaround time (TAT) as physicians had to send these tests out to other laboratories. Yet there is no evidence that patients are not receiving necessary laboratory tests or that any speculative increase in TAT has had a negative effect on patient outcomes.

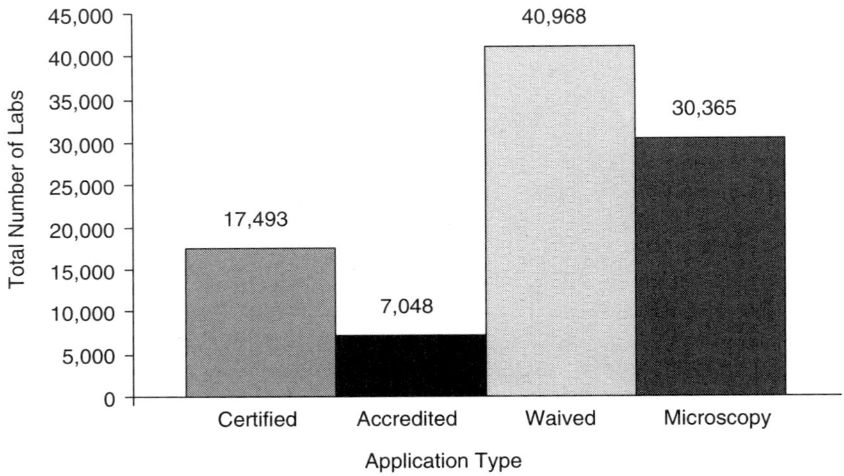

FIGURE 2.10 Physician office laboratories under CLIA by certification type, 1999. Note: Total number of POLs registered = 96,701. SOURCE: Health Care Financing Administration CLIA database (July 1999).

solidation discussed in the final section of this chapter. A 1995 OIG report analyzed the impact of CLIA on the availability of clinical laboratory services (OIG, 1995). The OIG tracked the volume, type, and frequency of laboratory tests provided to Medicare patients between 1985 and 1993 and analyzed data from a 1 percent sample of claims extracted annually from HCFA's Common Working File and its predecessor, the Part B Medicare Annual Data file. In order to learn more about CLIA's effect on physician practices, the OIG collected and analyzed survey data from physicians, including those in rural practices that had discontinued providing clinical laboratory services. Although hospital outpatient data are incomplete, the OIG found continued growth in the overall volume of tests, the number of tests per patient, and expenditures for clinical laboratory services since the implementation of CLIA in 1992. Additionally, the OIG found that CLIA does not appear to have affected physicians' ability to secure laboratory services for their patients. The OIG concluded that the 1988 amendments have not impaired the availability of laboratory services.

The CDC has requested comments on whether CLIA should be expanded to address the unique informed consent, ethical, and quality issues raised by genetic testing (Notice of Intent, 2000). This request is in response to studies that indicate a need to improve laboratory genetic testing practices and coordination between the laboratory, care provider, genetic counselor, and patient. The likely effect of an expanded CLIA on the cost of providing genetic testing is unknown.

CLIA's Impact on Quality

Data indicate sharp increases in both PT performance and CLIA laboratory registration rates from 1995 to 1996. CLIA requires PT for 86 tests or analytes.[18] Data show that in 1996, 87.4 percent of the scores from enrolled laboratories demonstrated no failures on PT[19], compared to 69.4 percent in 1995 (HCFA, 2000b). PT results from previously unregulated laboratories, particularly POLs, are most likely to be unacceptable (MMWR, 1996; Stull et al., 1998). The data also indicate that 93.2 percent of the laboratories required to be enrolled in PT were actually enrolled in 1996, compared to 89.6 percent in 1995. HCFA's target for fiscal year (FY) 1999 was that 90 percent of the scores for all 86 analytes requiring PT reported from all laboratories enrolled in PT should contain no failures and that 95 percent of all eligible laboratories would be participating.

Occupational Safety and Health Administration

Occupational Safety and Health Administration (OSHA) regulations protect the safety of workers, but also increase the cost of providing laboratory services. They touch almost every aspect of the provision of laboratory services. For instance, to minimize the transmission of infectious disease, health care workers and laboratory personnel are required to wear personal protective equipment (PPE) and to dispose of needles and other contaminated materials in specific ways. OSHA may require the use of "safety needles" in the future. Health care facilities, including physician offices, are required to have an occupational expo-

---

[18]This list of 86 analytes is made up largely of commonly performed diagnostic tests whose results are important in health care treatment decisions. Each laboratory performs PT on the regulated analytes that are a part of its specific test menu. There are other tests performed by laboratories, regulated under CLIA, for which PT is not required. Some of these tests are laboratory examinations and procedures that are so simple and accurate there is almost no likelihood of producing erroneous results. There are other tests for which PT is not yet available or may not yet be required by CLIA regulations. Some laboratories voluntarily participate in any PT that is available, even if not yet required under CLIA regulations. If no PT is available, laboratories are still supposed to take steps to validate their procedures. Tests for which PT is required may be added as CDC and HCFA update CLIA regulations (HCFA, 1998). PT does not evaluate errors made during the preanalytic or postanalytic phase of testing.

[19]Each laboratory is given 5 samples for each analyte. This is called a testing event. In most cases, the laboratory must obtain a satisfactory score on 4 out of 5 of these samples (80 percent). Some analytes such as blood type and Rh require 100 percent accuracy. A laboratory that is within the satisfactory range for all analytes is said to have no failures. Some analytes have fixed criteria to determine whether the laboratory was within a satisfactory range. For instance, on a serum cholesterol test, the laboratory is permitted to be within +/- 10 percent of the actual value. Other types of analytes are graded on a bell-shaped curve. The criteria for a satisfactory value for each analyte are outlined in 42CFR493 subpart H 493.821 of the CLIA regulations.

sure control plan. Contaminated waste, including leftover specimen samples, must be disposed of in a way that is more costly than disposal of regular trash. In addition, the transportation of certain human tissues and body fluids requires special packaging to protect the handler.[20] Each laboratory is required to develop a chemical hygiene plan which addresses the specific hazards found in its location and its approach to them (OSHA, 2000). Laboratories must also be equipped with proper ventilation to ensure safe air quality within the building (OSHA, 1999).

There are few data on the cost of compliance with OSHA regulations for the laboratory industry; however, tighter regulatory control usually means an increased financial and administrative burden. This burden has likely affected hospital-based, independent, and physician office laboratories and has implications for the cost of providing laboratory services.

MINIMIZING FRAUD, WASTE, AND ABUSE

The administration and Congress have tried to ensure that public funds are not wasted or abused by limiting physicians' ability to refer patients to a laboratory in which they have a financial interest, by aggressively investigating certain billing practices, and by denying payment for Medicare claims that are not deemed medically necessary.

Stark Amendments

The Ethics in Patient Referral Act (1998), commonly referred to as the Stark Amendments,[21] prohibits physicians from referring patients to laboratories and other designated health services in which they or their immediate family members have a financial interest.[22] It also attaches civil penalties to entities receiving these inappropriate referrals if they bill Medicare or Medicaid. The main purpose of the law is to reduce the overuse of health care services that can occur when physicians have a financial incentive to refer patients for laboratory services. A previous Institute Of Medicine (IOM) report showed that physicians order more laboratory tests when they profit from laboratory services (Gray, 1986).

Implementation of the Stark Amendments has been controversial (Committee urges final rule on Stark self-referral law revisions, 1999). Because Stark II was so broad, Congress added a number of exemptions to the rule that allow physicians to operate in-office laboratories and permit referrals made within certain types of "group practices" (Kalb, 1999). Several of the law's re-

---

[20]New CDC and Department of Transportation requirements may be imposed on packaging of diagnostic specimens.

[21]Named after the legislation's sponsor, Representative F. Pete Stark.

[22]The original legislation, or Stark I, enacted in 1989, restricted self-referral to laboratories. Stark II, enacted in 1993, expanded the statute to include 10 additional "designated health services."

quirements, however, raise concerns for physicians. For example, one of the requirements is that the physician or another member of the group must directly supervise the laboratory test. Direct supervision is more stringent than CLIA requirements because it means that the prescribing physician (or another physician member of the group) must be on site and immediately available during testing. There is anecdotal evidence that many laboratories are not aware of this requirement and, therefore, are not complying with its provisions. This is important because "the Stark laws contain no express requirement of intent; a physician can violate them even if he or she does not have any improper goal or purpose" (Kalb, 1999).

The Stark regulations also created a situation where independent physicians could no longer share laboratory facilities. Before these regulations, laboratories were commonly shared by independent practitioners to minimize expenses and provide a wider range of services than would be possible for a solo physician. Physicians must now either divest or form bona fide group practices to comply with the regulation.

In response to widespread confusion and public comment, HCFA attempted to clarify Stark II in a proposed rule (Proposed Rule, 1998). Because there was so much controversy and public comment in reaction to the proposed rule, the final rule has not been issued. HCFA is expected to issue a final rule later this year (Graziano, 2000). Several members of Congress have introduced legislation to bring the supervision requirement more in line with CLIA, but Congress has not acted on these proposals.

OIG Investigations

Spurred by concern during the last decade that laboratories were improperly billing the federal government, the OIG has conducted several major investigations that have resulted in significant settlements against providers of clinical laboratory services. These settlements have amounted to almost $1 billion dollars in recoveries, fines, and penalties (Grob, 2000). The OIG asserted that some laboratories were charging individually for tests that should have been billed as a panel at a lower rate (unbundling), using diagnosis codes that were never provided by a physician, providing kickbacks to physicians for patient referrals, double billing, and billing for unordered tests and tests that were not medically necessary (Grob, 2000). As a result of these cases, some laboratories not only paid large fines, but also signed agreements with the OIG called Corporate Integrity Agreements. The OIG has developed model compliance plans designed to assist clinical laboratories in developing internal controls that help prevent fraud, abuse, and waste (OIG, 2000).

Medical Necessity Review

In addition to retrospective reviews conducted by the OIG, Medicare contractors routinely review claims for certain tests against local medical criteria regarding the appropriateness of performing a particular test on a particular patient. This review is called local medical review policy (LMRP). Claims for laboratory tests that do not have a diagnosis code that is deemed to justify performance of the test may be denied even though the laboratory has no control over tests ordered by physicians. Contractors may also target certain providers, who have a history of inappropriate billing, for routine review.

Laboratory representatives testified that judgments regarding the medical appropriateness of laboratory tests, which are based solely on the presence or absence of particular International Classification of Diseases, Ninth Revision (ICD-9) diagnosis codes provided by the ordering physician, result in many inappropriate denials and a large administrative burden. The committee found a high rate of denials for some laboratory claims (Appendix E), but it was unable to determine what proportion of all outpatient laboratory claims were denied based on medical necessity criteria. HCFA data from 1998 showed that 12.3 percent of all POL claims were denied, but only 2.5 percent were denied because they were deemed medically unnecessary.

Appeals of denied claims are often expensive and time consuming. They also require participation of the physician who has little incentive to follow through. As a result, laboratory representatives testified that the current approach to assessment of medical necessity is misguided and results in an unfair financial burden on clinical laboratories.

PAYMENT TRENDS

Medicare payment trends for both inpatient and outpatient services, as well as some shift to capitated payments by both public and private payers, have squeezed the profit margins of the laboratory industry and limited the industry's ability to shift costs from payer to payer and test to test.

Medicare Shift to Prospective Payment Systems

A 1983 revision in Medicare payment policy for inpatient hospital services radically altered financial incentives for hospital laboratory services. Specifically, Medicare shifted from a reasonable cost reimbursement to a per-case approach based on diagnosis-related groups (DRGs).[23] The prospectively set payment amount was based on adjusted average historical costs and covers all services provided during the patient's stay. As a result, some cases may cost the hospital more than the Medicare payment, whereas other cases cost less. The system is designed to give hospitals an incentive to manage care more effi-

[23] Other third-party payers may pay on a per diem basis or negotiated rates.

ciently. Because of this change in payment policy, inpatient hospital laboratory testing became a cost center for Medicare patients rather than a profit center. The new payment policy thus created an incentive to reduce the number of tests ordered for hospital inpatients and to shift inpatient care to the outpatient setting.

The 1997 BBA mandated a change in the Medicare payment methodology for outpatient hospital services. Beginning in 2000, payments for outpatient services were also to be based on prospectively determined rates for bundled services. Clinical laboratory services provided under the clinical laboratory fee schedule are excluded from this change in payment methodology; however, significant payment policy changes were made in the way independent laboratories will be paid for pathology services. If a test is performed by an independent laboratory for a hospital outpatient department, the laboratory must bill the hospital for the technical component.[24] The hospital recoups what it pays the laboratory in the bundled payment amount it receives for the outpatient service. Previously, the laboratory was able to bill Medicare directly for the technical component (College of American Pathologists, 2000). Implementation of this billing requirement was recently delayed due to an intense lobbying effort by independent laboratories and the College of American Pathologists. Any major change in payment policy has the potential to affect the financial stability of the provider organization (in this case, hospitals) and to alter payment incentive structures for the provision of care.

Growth of Managed Care

The growth in managed care for both public and private payers has resulted in reduced revenue for the clinical laboratory industry.[25] Managed care organizations are typically defined as any third-party payer that uses cost-control or utilization-control mechanisms to direct the use of health care services. Almost all third-party payers now use managed care techniques to control costs. These techniques have reduced payments to laboratories and limited their ability to offset the cost of uncompensated services for patients who are uninsured, have limited coverage, or have coverage with particularly low payment rates.[26]

---

[24]The PPRC (1995) defines "technical component" as the part of a relative value or fee for a diagnostic test or therapeutic procedure that represents the cost of performing the service excluding the physician's work. The "professional component" is defined as the part of a relative value or fee that represents the cost of a physician's interpretation of a diagnostic test or treatment planning for a therapeutic procedure. Under this policy change, the independent laboratory is still permitted to bill Medicare directly for the professional component.

[25]According to a 1998 report by Interstudy, enrollment in the most aggressive type of managed care plan, health maintenance organizations, more than doubled, from 33.3 million to 81.3 million members, from 1990 to 1999.

[26]Medicaid payment rates are typically lower than those of other third-party payers.

Because of their ability to negotiate volume discounts, managed care organizations commonly pay significantly lower fees than other payers for laboratory services. In addition, many managed care plans pay laboratories on a capitated basis (Hoerger et al., 1996). Under a capitated payment arrangement, a laboratory is paid a fixed amount per member per month to provide all or a specified range of laboratory services for an enrolled population. Unlike the situation in which physicians or health maintenance organizations (HMOs) receive capitated payments for provision of care to patients, independent laboratories have little control over the volume or type of laboratory tests that are ordered and covered by the capitation rate.

Capitation of laboratory services first began in the mid-1990s and by the end of 1998 accounted for 20–25 percent of testing volume at the three largest national independent laboratories (Klipp, 2000). Driven in large part by their fear of losing market share, some hospitals and independent laboratories aggressively cut prices in bids for managed care contracts. Many laboratories bid below their costs in order to win capitated managed care contracts in the hope that physicians in the managed care plans would also use their services for non-managed care patients; however, there is little evidence that these "pull-through" expectations have been met (Hoerger et al., 1996; Klipp, 2000).

Managed care organizations generally prefer to contract with fewer laboratories that can provide services across larger geographic areas. The independent national and regional laboratories, therefore, were better positioned to provide services under capitated contracts, giving them an advantage over hospital-based laboratories; however, because of poorly negotiated managed care contracts, increased market share did not result in increased revenue for independent laboratories. In fact, according to Washington G-2 Reports, (Klipp, 2000) independent laboratories saw testing revenue drop from $10.4 billion to $8.1 billion, between 1993 and 1999, a decrease of 22 percent. This decline was due in part to poorly negotiated managed care contracts.

There appears to be a recent trend among independent laboratories to "walk away" from unprofitable managed care contracts. Laboratories may simply have learned from their mistakes, or mergers and acquisitions among the independent laboratories, discussed in more detail in the next section, may have given the largest laboratory companies the strength to pass up unfavorably priced contracts. Chief executive officers of the top independent laboratories have stated that they are beginning to focus less on volume and more on profitability (Klipp, 2000). In addition, it appears as though the growth in managed care may be slowing. The Lewin Group (2000) reports that consumers are shifting to more flexible plans; there is a growing backlash against managed care that has resulted in legislatively imposed coverage mandates, which in turn have reduced HMO profits. A recent survey from the American Association of Health Plans reports that many third-party payers are dropping their contracts to provide Medicare+Choice plans, Medicare's version of managed care (Morgan, 2000).

RESPONSE FROM THE INDUSTRY TO ENVIRONMENTAL TRENDS

The clinical laboratory industry has become very competitive despite the high degree of consolidation that has occurred in the independent laboratory sector. Changes in Medicare payment methodology, cuts in payment rates by Medicare and other payers, and the growth of managed care contracting have caused some laboratories, particularly hospital-based laboratories, to look to new markets in order to maintain profitability. These changes also have led to consolidation in both the independent and the hospital-based segments of the laboratory industry. In addition, hospital-based laboratories and independent laboratories have become engaged in head-to-head competition for market share as they strive to achieve levels of efficiency and critical mass that will allow them to compete effectively for outpatient, physician, and managed care business.

Market Consolidation and Network Development

Market consolidation has radically changed the face of the independent laboratory sector. In 1990, no single laboratory company had a major market share; rather, the eight largest companies accounted for 47 percent of the nationwide independent laboratory market (Hoerger et al., 1996). By 1999, two companies, Quest Diagnostics and LabCorp, largely through mergers and acquisitions, accounted for 61 percent of the testing conducted by independent laboratories (Klipp, 2000).

Some experts have raised concerns about the level of concentration in two national independent laboratories and the implications of that for industry competition. In the 1990s, laboratory consolidation was viewed as conferring an advantage for negotiating managed care contracts. Although two companies now dominate the independent laboratory market with an estimated 61 percent of total test volume, that is only 16 percent of the total clinical laboratory market share, including hospital-based and physicians' office laboratories.

Hospitals also have responded to the changing health care marketplace by forming regional laboratory networks with other hospitals and independent laboratories. This consolidation began in earnest in the mid-1990s with the formation of integrated delivery systems. Networks have taken different approaches to how they consolidate their laboratories (including intralaboratory, interlaboratory, intrahospital, and interhospital consolidation), but they also have tried to reduce costs by increasing operational efficiencies (Farwell, 1995).

Some in the industry believe that hospital-based laboratories have an advantage over independent laboratories in the current environment (Steiner and Root, 1999). Hospitals are better situated than most commercial laboratories to provide STAT (literally, at once) testing and same-day test results. At the same time, commercial laboratories may be better positioned, in terms of the types of testing they do, to incorporate newer, more complex tests.

TABLE 2.6 Hospital Laboratory Outpatient–Outreach Test Volume as a Percentage of Total Hospital Testing, Selected Years

Staffed Acute Care Beds	1987	1991	1993	1996	1998
150–300	25.8	30.6	38.0	40.9	42.8
>300	23.2	26.9	31.6	37.2	35.0

SOURCE: Klipp, 2000.

Growth of Hospital-Based Laboratory Outreach Programs

During the 1990s, because of changes in inpatient payment policy (described above), hospitals shifted a great deal of inpatient services to the outpatient setting. To make up for the inpatient volume that was lost to nonhospital laboratories providing tests to outpatients, hospitals have developed outreach programs to bring testing into their laboratories from physicians outside the hospital.

Since the early 1990s, the average number of inpatient tests per discharge has declined, while outpatient test volume has grown as a percentage of total hospital-based testing. Table 2.6 presents outpatient and outreach volume as a percentage of total hospital-based testing since 1987. Change has been most significant in the 150- to 300-bed hospitals, with outpatient and outreach volume as a percentage of total hospital testing increasing almost 66 percent from 1987 to 1998. For hospitals with more than 300 beds, the increase over the same period was almost 51 percent.

While volume has been growing, revenue per outreach test has been shrinking. Washington G-2 Reports (Klipp, 2000) estimates that from 1994 to 1999, revenue per outreach test decreased from $16.50 to $11.50, a decline of more than 30 percent. Hospitals in areas of high managed care penetration have seen outreach test revenue decline even further, to less than $10 per test.

SUMMARY

The laboratory industry is composed of hospital-based, independent, and physician office laboratories. The industry appears to be both resilient and vulnerable to environmental trends. For instance, after being hit hard by global trends toward managed care and cost containment, the two largest independent laboratories not only have survived, but are rebounding. Hospital-based laboratories have been able to increase their outpatient and outreach business in response to declines in inpatient business. The numbers of POLs initially declined in response to federal regulatory policies designed to improve the quality of laboratory testing but are now increasing, partially in response to an increase in the number of waived tests available. Overall, test volume is up, but revenue per test and aggregate Medicare Part B spending for outpatient laboratory services are down.

Many factors have affected the cost of providing laboratory services. New regulatory requirements have increased the cost of doing business; however, the industry has also found ways to reduce costs through consolidation that provides economies of scale. Demand for laboratory services is likely to grow as the population ages and innovation makes new tests possible.

In many laboratories, innovative technologies and increased regulatory requirements have reduced the length of time it takes for the physician to receive laboratory test results and have improved quality and patient convenience. Improved quality has been demonstrated through proficiency testing. An increase in the number of waived tests has made it easier for patients to undergo testing during a visit to the doctor. In addition to being more convenient for patients, testing closer to the physician leads to faster turnaround time that may speed diagnosis and treatment.

Environmental trends, particularly payment trends, have the potential to affect beneficiary access to laboratory testing. Coding, coverage, and payment problems, such as delays in assigning codes to new technology and the current approach to determining medical necessity that leads to inappropriate denials, could create barriers to beneficiary access to care.

REFERENCES

Auxter, S. 1999. Are physician office laboratories making a comeback? *Clinical Laboratory News*, March.

Binns, H. J., S. LeBailly, and H. G. Gardner. 1998. The physicians' office laboratory: 1988 and 1996 survey of Illinois pediatricians. Pediatric Practice Research Group [see comments]. *Arch Pediatr Adolesc Med* 152, No. 6:585–592. Comment in: *Arch Pediatr Adolesc Med* 1998; 152, No. 12:1248–1249.

Bogdanich, W. November 2, 1987a. Lax laboratories: The Pap test misses much cervical cancer through labs' errors. *Wall Street Journal*.

Bogdanich, W. December 29, 1987b. Physicians' carelessness with Pap tests is cited in procedure's high volume failure rate. *Wall Street Journal*.

Boone, D. J. 1992. Literature review of research related to the Clinical Laboratory Improvement Amendments of 1988 [see comments]. *Arch Pathol Lab Med* 116, No. 7: 681–693. Comment in: *Arch Pathol Lab Med* 1992; 116, No. 7:679–680.

Born, P. H., and S. L. Thran. 1998. The influence of CLIA '88 on physician office laboratories. *J Fam Pract* 46, No. 4:319–327.

Centers for Disease Control and Prevention (CDC) 1995. *Clinical Laboratory Improvement Committee Summary Report*. Atlanta, GA: CDC.

CDC. 2000. CLIA Waived Test List. Web page accessed August 3, 2000. Available at http://www.phppo.cdc.gov/dls/clia/waived.asp.

Chapin, K., and E. J. Baron. 1995. Impact of CLIA 88 on the clinical microbiology laboratory. *Diagn Microbiol Infect Dis* 23, No. 1–2:35–43.

College of American Pathologists. 2000. Hospital Outpatient PPS Information for Pathologists. Web page accessed August 4, 2000. Available at http://www.cap.org/html/advocacy/capdocs/pps.html.

Committee urges final rule on Stark self-referral law revisions. June 7, 1999. *AMA News*.

Donaldson, Lufkin & Jenrette. 1993. *Laboratory Services—Independent Clinical Laboratories*. New York, NY: Donaldson, Lufkin & Jenrette.

Dyckman, Z., and B. B. Cassidy. 2000. Recent Developments and Trends in the Clinical Laboratory Industry (unpublished). Columbia, MD.

Ethics in Patient Referral Act. 1998. 42 USC 1385nn.

Farwell, D. C. 1995. Hospital laboratory consolidation. Reduce costs, improve service, enhance the workplace. *Clin Lab Manage Rev* 9, No. 5:411–420.

Gray, B. H. 1986. *For-Profit Enterprise in Health Care*. Washington, DC: National Academy Press.

Graziano, C. July 2000. "Stark II" rule expected soon. *CAP Today,* p. 116.

Grob, G. January 20, 2000. Testimony before the IOM Committee on Medicare Payment Methodology for Clinical Laboratory Services: Medicare payments for clinical laboratory services: Vulnerabilities and controls. Washington, DC.

Gustafson, T. January 20, 2000. Testimony before the IOM Committee on Medicare Payment Methodology for Clinical Laboratory Services. Washington, DC.

Guterman, S. 2000. Putting Medicare in Context: How Does the Balanced Budget Act Affect Hospitals? (unpublished). Washington, DC: The Urban Institute.

Health Care Financing Administration (HCFA). 1998. CLIA: General Program Description. Web page, accessed February 17, 2000. Available at www.hcfa.gov/medicaid/clia/progdesc.htm.

HCFA. 2000a. *March 2000 CLIA Provider Files, Reported Annual Test Volume*.

HCFA. 2000b. CLIA Performance Goal in HCFA's Annual Performance Plan: Improve Laboratory Testing Accuracy. Web page accessed July 11, 2000. Available at http://www.hcfa.gov/medicaid/clia/perfmeas.htm.

Hoerger, T. J., J. L. Eggleston, and R. C. Lindrooth. 1996. *Background Report on the Clinical Laboratory Industry, Draft Report.* Research Triangle Park, NC.

Inhorn, S. L., J. E. Shalkham, and G. B. Mueller. 1994. Quality assurance programs to meet CLIA requirements. *Diagn Cytopathol* 11, No. 2:195–200.

Kalb, P. E. 1999. Health care fraud and abuse. *JAMA* 282, No. 12:1163–1168.

Klipp, J. 2000. *Lab Industry Strategic Outlook 2000: Market Trends & Analysis*. Washington, DC: Washington G-2 Reports.

Lehman Brothers. 1993. *Corning: Trying to Get Comfortable with the Clinical Lab Business*. New York, NY: Lehman Brothers.

Levit, K., C. Cowan, H. Lazenby, A. Sensenig, et al., 2000. Health spending in 1998: Signals of change. *Health Affairs*. 19, No. 1: 124–132.

Lewin Group. 2000. *Outlook for Medical Technology Innovation: Will Patients Get the Care They Need? Report 1: The State of the Industry*. Washington, DC: Health Industry Manufacturers Association.

Merrill Lynch. 1999. *Quest Diagnostics: Leader in Sector with Improving Fundamentals*, reference # 60126501. New York: Merril Lynch.

Morbidity and Mortality Weekly Report (MMWR). March 8, 1996. Clinical laboratory performance on proficiency test samples—United States, 1994. 45, No. 9: 193–196.

Morgan, D. June 30, 2000. More health plans quit Medicare. *Washington Post,* section A, p. 8.

Notice of Intent; Genetic testing under the Clinical Laboratory Improvement Amendments. 2000. *Federal Register* 65, No. 87:25928–25934.

Office of the Inspector General (OIG). 1995. *CLIA's Impact on the Availability of Laboratory Services*. Washington, DC: OIG.

OIG. 2000. Corporate Integrity Agreements (CIAs) and Settlement Agreements with Integrity Provisions. Web page accessed September 5, 2000. Available at http://www.dhhs.gov/oig/cia/index.htm.

Occupational Safety and Health Administration (OSHA). 1999. Ventilation. Web page accessed July 12, 2000. Available at http://www.osha-slc.gov/SLTC/ventilation/index.html.

OSHA. 2000. Laboratories. Web page accessed July 12, 2000. Available at http://www.osha-slc.gov/SLTC/laboratories/index.html.

Physician Payment Review Commission (PPRC). 1995. *Annual Report to Congress*, 1995. Washington, DC: PPRC.

Proposed Rule: Physicians' referrals to health care entities with which they have financial relationships. 1998. *Federal Register* 63, No. 6:1659–1728.

Rej, R., and R. W. Jenny. 1992. How good are clinical laboratories? An assessment of current performance [published erratum appears in *Clin Chem* 1993; 39, No. 3:558]. *Clin Chem* 38, No. 7:1210–1217; discussion 1218–1225.

Roussel, P. L. 1996. Impact of CLIA on physician office laboratories in rural Washington State [published erratum appears in *J Fam Pract* 1997; 44, No. 2:214]. *J Fam Pract* 43, No. 3:249–254.

Smith Barney Research. 1990. *The Clinical Laboratory Industry, Investment Outlook.* New York, NY: Smith Barney.

Steiner, J. W., and J. M. Root. June 1999. The battle between hospital and commercial labs: Who's winning? *Clinical Laboratory News,* p. 4.

Strauss, S., G. S. Cembrowski, and S. A. Adlis. 1995. CLIA's effect on POLs (physicians' office laboratories). *MLO Med Lab Obs* 27, No. 6:34–38.

Stull, T. M., Hearn, T. L., Hancock, J. S., Handsfield, J. H. et al., 1998. Variation in proficiency testing performance by testing site. *JAMA* 279, No. 6: 463–467.

3
Technology Trends in the Clinical Laboratory Industry

The laboratory environment has been characterized by ongoing rapid and dramatic innovation since the 1980s. There has been remarkable growth in the range and complexity of available tests and services, which is expected to continue. Laboratory technology is often at the forefront of medical advances. In some cases, testing techniques to diagnose or screen for a particular condition are available before effective treatment. Innovation in laboratory technology, which includes both new tests and advances in equipment and testing techniques, has made testing more efficient and automated. Information technology (IT) has revolutionized the transfer of data by decreasing the time it takes to order and receive test results and by creating opportunities for research on large datasets. Many predict that clinical laboratory technology will play an even more important role in the future delivery of health care (Felder et al., 1999; Wilkinson, 1997). Innovation in health care, particularly when it is more efficient than existing methods (see Box 3.1), is welcomed by payers, providers, and patients; however, the efficient integration of innovation into medical care may be affected by policies related to coverage, coding, and payment.

There are wide variations in the types of technology employed by different types of laboratories. The discussion of technology trends below does not mean that these trends are occurring in all settings. For example, certain small laboratories do not have the volume of testing to justify automated or elaborate IT systems.

This chapter reviews the three major technological innovations that have radically altered the way samples are collected and analyzed and the way results

BOX 3.1 The Future of Technology

Edwina Clark, a 42 year old woman with diabetes, no longer needs to test her blood sugar concentrations every day because she now has a glucose sensor implanted under the skin of her thigh. Her toilet at home provides a double check because it can analyze glucose, protein, and bacteria concentrations in her urine. Instead of giving herself daily injections of insulin, she now relies on an implanted insulin reservoir that automatically adjusts her insulin dose. Her blood sugar concentrations are so well controlled that she is unlikely ever to develop any of the vascular and neurological complications that used to be common.

This futuristic case was taken directly from a 1999 editorial in the *British Medical Journal* (Berger and Smith, 1999).

are reported. These innovations include automation, IT, and laboratory measurement or testing technology. The changes that these technological developments produce, especially how and where testing services are delivered and laboratory-staffing needs, are also discussed.

AUTOMATION

Automation has been, and promises to continue to be, an important force in the changing laboratory marketplace. Laboratory automated (and manual) processes occur in three stages:

1. ***Preanalytic stage:*** This includes, choosing the test, placing the order, preparing the patient, collecting the specimen, transporting the specimen, any specimen preparation work, and daily quality controls.
2. ***Analytic stage:*** This involves actual testing of the specimen and all routine procedures up to result reporting.
3. ***Postanalytic stage:*** This is concerned primarily with forwarding results to the appropriate hospital department or physician and routine daily maintenance and shutdown (Travers and Krochmal, 1988).[1]

[1]The three stages of clinical laboratory testing, specifically within the laboratory, were defined in 1988 by Eleanor Travers and Charles Krochmal. Others categorize the computer entry of demographics, test request review, and specimen preparation, including specimen labeling and centrifugation, as a part of the analytic rather than the preanalytic phase of testing (Cruse, 1998). Still others would include steps that take place in the doctor's office prior to placing the order and following delivery of the test results within these phases.

Preanalytic Stage

Although some progress has been made in automating the preanalytic phase of testing, much of the work in this phase is still performed manually. In some settings, such as within the hospital, specimens are transferred efficiently using a pneumatic tubing system. In an independent laboratory setting, specimens are often transported manually by courier to the testing site.[2] In most settings of care, specimens are collected and labeled with identifying information and are entered into the laboratory computer system manually. In addition, most decisions about the adequacy of the specimen's volume and whether the specimen is in the correct type of container are made by a laboratory technician, not a machine (McPherson, 1998).

There are many opportunities to automate preanalytic processes. For instance, specimen containers can be prelabeled with bar codes that link specimens to identifying electronic information. The container may also contain substances that automatically prepare the sample for processing (Felder et al., 1999). There has been progress with optical character recognition hardware and software that can "read" labels (Burtis, 1996). Test tubes may eventually have computer chips embedded in the stopper (Felder et al., 1999). Technology to automate many of the processes for aliquot[3] or specimen preparation, sample quality testing, specimen transport and handling, and automatic accessioning[4] exist but are not widely used (McPherson, 1998). Test ordering over the Internet may increase efficiency and reduce administrative errors during specimen collection and processing. Machines eventually may draw blood specimens, and robots may transport specimens from hospitalized patients to the hospital laboratory (Felder et al., 1999; Wilkinson, 1997).

Analytic Stage

In most laboratory settings, the analytic stage of testing is more automated. Beginning in the 1960s, several rounds of sophisticated automation resulted in multianalyzers, which are multichannel instruments that measure many different analytes.[5] Automative technology also allows groups of tests, called "panels" or "profiles," to be run on the same sample. A similar evolution occurred in the hematology laboratory, where the counting of different types of blood cells is consolidated and expanded to include automated differentials on the same in-

---

[2]While transport is still manual, the development of a global transportation system that facilitates rapid transport of people and goods has enabled independent laboratories to centralize their facilities and reduce costs through economies of scale (Burtis, 1996).

[3]An aliquot is the small portion of a specimen taken for an assay or test.

[4]Accession is the process of identifying a specimen and entering a unique specimen identifier into laboratory records.

[5]An analyte is any substance that is measured. The term is usually applied to a component of blood or other body fluid.

strument (McPherson, 1998). A chemistry, hematology, coagulation, or urinalysis analyzer can now generate highly precise and accurate results in only a few minutes (Cruse, 1998).

Consolidation of tests and testing equipment is possible in part because operator activities for each type of test are interchangeable. Running tests is simplified by redesigning equipment ("analyzers") to look and function similarly on the outside, even though very different operations are done inside. According to Richard McPherson, "The tasks that attendant operators conduct now (sample presentation, result review, and quality control) are quite similar on very different analyzers" (McPherson, 1998).

Emerging in the early 1980s, consolidated workstations contain several instruments in one area. Typically, the area is managed by one technical person supervising several nontechnical staff (Cruse, 1998).[6] The technical staff member monitors all instruments, and reviews and releases the test results (McPherson, 1998). The workstation approach increases the productivity of the laboratory, reduces personnel costs, and dramatically decreases testing turnaround time (TAT) (Cruse, 1998).

Modular laboratory automation was introduced during the 1990s and represents a more sophisticated design than approaches aimed at automating the entire laboratory all at once. This technology permits the laboratory to begin with a basic configuration and add automated modules as needed. Thus, a laboratory can buy only the modular pieces that best meet its needs. It also makes integrating the new technology into existing laboratory architecture easier because the modular units are small and mobile (Sainato, 2000). Only a few vendors of modular automation are in the market at this time (Marietti, 1998). Robots may be part of a facility's modular laboratory automation system. Although especially beneficial for tasks such as serology, blood grouping, and tissue typing, (Lifshitz and De Cresce, 1989), robots are not used as extensively by the clinical laboratory industry in the United States as they are in Japan.[7]

Replacing manual steps with automated processes virtually eliminated the risk of mistakes and reduced testing error rates (Howanitz, 1994). Enhancements in automated processing resulted in improved technical precision and accuracy. According to McPherson (1998), "the vast majority of assays demonstrate technical variabilities that are well within medical needs."

---

[6]When considering the task conducted by individuals who do not have technical skills, it is important to note that many states have licensure laws that preclude the conduct of certain testing procedures by nontechnical staff. In addition, Clinical Laboratory Improvement Amendments of 1988 requirements, as they relate to moderate- and high-complexity tests, do not allow the use of nontechnical staff for certain testing procedures.

[7]Japan is more focused on industrial robotics in general and chose to make the investment in laboratory robotics. Laboratories in the United States have been slower to adopt this technology because of its high cost and difficulty integrating it into existing laboratory architecture.

Postanalytic Stage

Over the past 20 years, the postanalytic phase has become more automated. In the 1980s, test results were often transferred by courier or mail. In the 1990s, they were sometimes conveyed over the telephone or via fax. Today, in some laboratories, the completed results are automatically forwarded to the appropriate area of the hospital or physician office electronically through the use of dedicated printers, and billing and utilization report generation is computerized (McPherson, 1998). Use of the Internet to report results would likely reduce costs by eliminating the need for designated fax and telephone lines. In addition, quicker TAT may lead to reduced episode-of-care costs.

Many analytic and postanalytic tasks are now automated using process control software (Markin and Whalen, 2000). For instance, repeat, reflex, [8] and add-on [9] testing are managed through electronic systems.[10] Electronic systems may also manage specimen transportation, storage, and disposal. Finally, these systems monitor consistency of results and ensure that panic values are called to medical staff's attention.

Billing and collection processes may become more automated in the future. Laboratories may automatically obtain and transmit all required documentation necessary for payers to process the claim through electronic systems (e.g., patient's name, address, and primary and secondary insurance information). Additional information required includes referring provider information, the patient's copay responsibilities, diagnosis codes, and other data that might be necessary to demonstrate medical necessity. Typically this information is transmitted manually each time a test is ordered. Integrating electronic systems that automatically send updated information electronically every time a test is ordered would increase efficiency.

There are steps that take place after the laboratory submits its results to the physician including physician interpretation and physician and patient action. After physicians receive the results, they must interpret what those results mean for the patient. Sometimes the physician is assisted in interpreting results by normal ranges included in the laboratory report or a written explanation of the testing results. In some cases, the physician may consult with a laboratorian to better understand the meaning of the test results. The next step is the physician's course of action. The laboratory tests may indicate that all test results are normal and that no action needs to be taken other than informing the patient of the results. Other courses of action might include additional laboratory testing, hospitalization, changing a medication or the dose of a medication, initiating a new course of treatment, monitoring the patient more closely, or counseling a patient to

[8]Reflex tests are tests that are reordered by a physician after an abnormal test result.

[9]Add-on tests are tests ordered on the same sample after the initial tests have been conducted.

[10]For Medicare payment policy, the Office of the Inspector General (OIG) spells out specific guidelines for reflex and add-on testing.

change certain health-related behaviors. The ultimate outcome for the patient is not simply dependent on obtaining an accurate test value. It also depends on the physician's interpretation and the action taken by both the physician and patient.

INFORMATION TECHNOLOGY

Like many other areas of healthcare delivery, laboratory services are experiencing an IT revolution. Laboratory experts that keep pace with emerging IT have found new, more efficient ways to communicate and provide services; educate themselves, their staff, and their clients; market their products; and manage data and information.

Because Internet-based communications are inexpensive and not hampered by time differences and geographic distance, experts predict that the Internet will become the primary means of communication in the future (Burtis, 1996; Klatt, 1997). Requests for testing and test results will be communicated electronically. Electronic image transmission will mean that hard-to-diagnose images can be sent quickly and efficiently to national specialty centers (Wilkinson, 1997). Test result reports will be linked to journal articles and other sophisticated multimedia information sources (Friedman, 1998). This capability may become more important with the increased use of genetic testing by general practitioners since physicians often do not understand the meaning of genetic test results (Holtzman, 1999). Streamlining the cost of providing this additional information will also be important since individual consults with a laboratory expert are often not paid for separately and must be worked into the cost of the test.

The use of electronic systems creates the opportunity to improve laboratory services. For instance, laboratory results for certain tests can be influenced by drug use. Patient records could include all pharmaceuticals the patient is taking. The computer could then be programmed to identify cases in which the results are likely to be affected, and it may even be able to assist in the interpretation of test results and suggest appropriate actions to be taken.

Internet-based reporting creates opportunities to communicate test results directly to patients. In the spring of 2000, Quest Diagnostics, a large national independent laboratory, began offering consumers direct access to test results via an Internet healthcare Web site owned by Caresoft, Inc., called "TheDailyApple.com." Only patients who are registered with TheDailyApple.com may access their data on-line. Their physicians will have the opportunity to review the results before information is put on-line. Only routine test results are offered, and Caresoft sends personal identification numbers to users via the U.S. mail to ensure confidentiality (Direct-to-consumer test result reporting, 2000). [11]

---

[11] In some states, providers, and patients may be prohibited from utilizing this type of Internet-based service. Most states have specific laws that address direct access to medical data within the context of a patient's rights to records. For example, by statute in Tennessee, a patient cannot access medical records directly. Other states' laws say that pa-

Information technology will change the way laboratorians educate themselves and their staff. Laboratory professionals can interact with one another through e-mail and specialized LISTSERVs (Burtis, 1996). They also have access to technical libraries in electronic format (Burtis, 1996). Experts predict that IT will radically alter the format and role of medical journals. They will be more electronically based with links to multimedia sources of information (Berger and Smith, 1999).

Information technology has created new marketing and advertising opportunities for laboratories (Klatt, 1997). Increased consumer empowerment, new testing techniques that are simple enough for home use or home sample collection, and IT have combined to create new direct-to-consumer marketing opportunities for laboratory tests. Laboratories may follow the pharmaceutical industry's lead by marketing directly to consumers and by making products directly available to consumers over the Internet. For instance, there is a consumer-based market for "drugs-of-abuse" tests, home-based HIV tests, glucose monitoring, pregnancy and ovulation tests, and genetic tests. Consumers may prefer to bypass their personal physician for convenience and to keep test results out of their medical records. Most of these types of tests are paid for by consumers, so they do not have the incentive of insurance coverage to obtain these tests through their health care provider.

Collecting and analyzing patient outcome data may become more essential in the marketing of laboratory services as third-party payers increasingly demand evidence that new health care services are cost-effective and positively affect patient outcomes. New hardware and software have increased the laboratory's ability to store and process data. Currently, Quest Diagnostics maintains the world's largest private database of clinical laboratory test results. It intends to use these resources to add value to its laboratory services (Where is the lab industry headed, 2000). For example, data may be used to track a patient's progress, minimize redundant testing, evaluate phlebotomists' collection technique, and track patient outcomes (McDonald, 1997; Plebani, 1999). Large databases can also be used to track disease outbreaks and conduct other types of public health research (McPherson, 1998). While research opportunities abound, laboratories will be challenged to identify ways to protect confidential patient information and obtain patients' informed consent to participate in research (Chou, 1996).

LABORATORY MEASUREMENT AND TESTING TECHNOLOGY

Laboratory testing technology advances through both incremental and breakthrough developments. Incremental changes often make testing processes simpler, more efficient (and often less expensive), and of higher quality. Less

---

tients may access their medical records only with the written permission of the ordering physician or by legal request.

frequently, technology makes major advances that result in totally new tests or testing techniques.

Esoteric Tests

Esoteric tests are relatively uncommon tests that are dependent on physician interpretation skill. As of the mid-1990s, approximately 1,250 different tests were performed by the clinical laboratory industry, about half of which were classified as "routine" (Smith Barney, 1995). For example, in the late 1980s, polymerase chain reaction (PCR) testing was "cutting-edge" technology. Today, PCR is very common and is used for approximately 165,000–220,000 viral load tests for HIV and hepatitis C each year (Klipp, 2000). Because PCR has become so common, it has lost its esoteric label.

The total U.S. market for esoteric testing is roughly $2 billion annually, for 50 million specimens (Klipp, 2000). In 1998, this market consisted of $1.4 billion in reference work for hospitals and $618 million in reference work for independent laboratories (Klipp, 2000).[12] The median price of tests sent out by hospitals declined 20 percent, from an estimated $28.73 per test in 1996 to $23.19 in 1998 (Klipp, 2000). With 1.4–1.8 tests performed on the average sample, the average revenue generated per specimen is between $33 and $42 (Klipp, 2000). As esoteric tests become more commonly performed, competition and economies of scale may increase, driving prices down further, even in the esoteric market.

Genetic Testing

With the mapping of the human genome, the field of molecular diagnostics, which includes genetic testing, is expected to grow rapidly during the next five years.[13] Genetic tests are able to detect gene mutations. Early detection may allow clinicians to predict predisposition to disease. This is important because genetics are possibly a significant factor in seven of the top ten causes of death in the United States (Klipp, 2000). In addition to addressing the factors associated with these causes of death, genetic testing is also used for determining HIV and hepatitis viral loads, making prenatal diagnoses, identifying chromosome abnormalities, determining the paternity of a child, ascertaining cancer cytogenetics, and identifying inherited or predisposition to diseases.

As of August 2000, an Internet-based directory of genetics laboratories reports that 469 laboratories and 895 genetic clinics in the United States were performing tests for 753 genetic diseases, compared to only 110 laboratories that conducted genetic tests for 111 different diseases in 1993 (Children's Health

---

[12]Reference work includes testing that is sent to an outside laboratory for completion. Many hospital-based, independent, and physician office laboratories do not have adequate equipment and personnel to conduct their own esoteric testing.

[13]Some experts believe that current expectations for genetic testing are overblown (Holtzman and Marteau, 2000; Jones, 2000).

Care System, 1999). Not all genetic tests are FDA approved for clinical use; some may be available only in a research setting.[14]

A future trend in genetic testing is a focus on prevention. According to Robert Nakamura, the emphasis will "shift from costly intervention and treatment of established diseases to proactive prediction and prevention of disease." He anticipates that predictive tests will screen for data identifying important population genetic risk factors for diabetes, cancer, and autoimmune diseases (Nakamura, 1999). Early identification of immunologic markers that predict autoimmune diseases may facilitate early intervention with autoantigen-specific therapy, targeted directly at the component of the immune system that causes disease (Nakamura, 1999). According to Nakamura, "This approach will require new information systems that will link large-scale databanks and special programs for data mining and retrieval in bioinformatics, cheminformatics, and population genetics. The clinical laboratory will soon be able to provide powerful new molecular diagnostic tools along with multianalytic assays for expression of genes and proteins in different patterns of diseases, disease progression, and predisposition to disease" (Nakamura, 1999).

Pharmacogenomics

More than 100,000 Americans die every year from side effects of properly prescribed medicines, and another 2 million are made seriously ill (Weiss, 2000). This occurs because medicines are made and sold on a standardized basis even though people vary substantially in the way they respond to these compounds. However, as scientists uncover more and more genes that control individual responses to medications, physicians should be able to base prescribing decisions on a patient's individual genetic makeup (Evans and Relling, 1999). The cost implications of this new science, called pharmacogenomics, are unclear. This type of genetic screening will likely increase the front-end cost of providing care. It could, however, result in better health outcomes and long-term cost savings substantial enough to offset the initial expense, particularly if

[14]Clinical tests are those in which specimens are examined and results reported to the provider and/or patient for the purpose of diagnosis, prevention, or treatment in the care of individual patients. U.S. laboratories performing clinical tests must be Clinical Laboratory Improvement Amendments (CLIA) approved. Research tests are those in which specimens are examined for the purpose of understanding a condition better or developing a clinical test. Test results are generally not given to patients or their providers. Rarely, a research laboratory will, at the patient's request, share potentially useful findings with a clinical laboratory so the patient's test results can be confirmed and a formal report issued. Laboratories performing research testing are not subject to CLIA regulation. The cost of research testing is generally covered by the researcher. Requests for participation in research may be denied, at the laboratory's discretion, if the laboratory has sufficient samples or the subject does not fit the research project goals.

screening efforts target subpopulations that are more likely to be susceptible to the genetic characteristic.

Nanotechnology

Nanotechnology, the science of building miniature devices out of very small particles such as individual atoms, molecules, viruses, or cells, merges biological and IT science. Nanotechnology has the potential to exponentially increase computer power through smaller, faster computer processors. Nanotechnology research could continue to expand during the coming years with a boost from President Clinton's 2001 budget, which proposes to create a National Nanotechnology Initiative. The President's proposal includes $495 million for research projects, an 83 percent increase over funding for this year. Seventy percent of the money will go to university-based research (Executive Office of the President, 2000; McGee, 2000).

Nanotechnology promises to affect the clinical laboratory industry through the development of miniaturized components and devices for chemical processing and measuring sensors (Burtis, 1996). This technology could prove to be extremely useful in the movement toward developing small, versatile point-of-care tests. According to Chad Mirkin, acting director for the Center for Nanofabrication and Molecular Assembly at Northwestern University, nanotechnology is already used in tests for tuberculosis and colon cancer (McGee, 2000). It has improved our ability to see chemical processes and microscopic structures in biological systems (Roco et al., 1999). Another potential application is in drug administration. Some drugs dissolve more easily if they are nanometersize (McGee, 2000). Although the potential of nanotechnology is substantial, a great deal of basic scientific research must be completed before clinical applications will be available.

TECHNOLOGY'S EFFECT ON SITE OF SERVICE

Some laboratory testing has moved out of the laboratory and is closer to the patient. Point-of-care testing (POCT) provides rapid test results within minutes of taking the sample, and home testing affords the ultimate consumer convenience, testing from the comfort of one's home. Experts disagree about whether this trend is the beginning of a dramatic shift in site of service for laboratory testing (Maibach et al., 1998; Woo and Henry, 1994). Although trend data show that these markets are growing, concerns about costs, the potential for errors, difficulties in linking test results to other clinical processes and information systems, and coverage restrictions by third-party payers may limit the growth of these two expanding testing markets (Sainato, 1999).

BOX 3.2 Point-of-Care Testing

"In just a few years, primary care physicians may be able to get a complete-blood count (CBC) for a patient simply by shining a light in the patient's eye or sticking a probe under the patient's tongue. This technology provides immediate test results, minimizes patient discomfort, reduces the risk of needle stick injuries, is free from concerns about contamination, eliminates the need to dispose of left-over blood samples, and is likely to be much less costly than traditional laboratory blood tests." SOURCE: (Uehling, 2000).

Point-of-Care Testing

New technologies not only have made POCT devices small and portable but also have improved specimen collection techniques so that they are minimally invasive. The relatively small size and user-friendly nature of this technology is due in large part to the advances in microprocessor-based analyzers and disposable test cartridges containing biosensor-laden silicon tests (Klipp, 2000). New laser-based skin perforators permit the collection of just a few microliters of interstitial fluid for testing glucose levels, and infrared sensors are being used to measure glucose and other analytes (e.g., bilirubin) directly through the skin (Felder et al., 1999). Multianalyte, spectroscopy-based, noninvasive sensors will provide a wide range of analytical tests at the bedside in the near future (Felder et al., 1999). Table 3.1 outlines certain POCT applications in 1999 and the estimated expenditures for each category.

Sales of POCT devices and tests to hospitals and physicians offices in the United States were roughly $1.1 billion in 1998, and nationwide. POCT expenditures are expected to grow at an average annual rate of 9 percent from 2000 to 2005 (Klipp, 2000). One industry expert suggests that 80 percent of laboratory testing will be available at the patient's bedside within the next five years at a fraction of the cost of centralized testing (Felder et al., 1999).

There is controversy over the cost-effectiveness of POCT versus centralized laboratory testing particularly since cost-effectiveness and patient outcomes data are lacking. Research from the early 1990s found that the cost per test using a POCT analyzer was significantly higher than central laboratory costs (Tsai et al., 1994). Others have found that not all types of POCT decrease the TAT of the entire diagnostic process, save sufficient amounts of money to justify the additional expense (Van Heyningen et al., 1999), or positively affect patient outcomes (Kendall et al., 1998; Parvin et al., 1996; Rose et al., 1997). These findings have led one expert to conclude that POCT will never become the primary mode of testing (Friedman, 1998). Others have found that under certain conditions, however, POCT can be provided at the same or lower cost than centralized services (Felder et al., 1999; Root, 1997). Since cost analysis methods have

TABLE 3.1 Point-of-Care Test Expenditures, 1999

Test Category	Expenditures ($ million)
Blood glucose	375
Blood gas [a]	262
Urine Strips, HCG	157
Electrolytes	137
Coagulation	70
Cholesterol	53
Infectious diseases	47

NOTE: HCG = human chorionic gonadotropin.

[a] Blood gas applications include the following five tests: (1) pH, the measurement of alkalinity in the blood; (2) Pco_2, the measurement of the partial pressure of carbon dioxide in the blood; (3) Hco^{-3}, the bicarbonate ion, which is a measurement of the metabolic (renal) component of the acid–base equilibrium; (4) Po_2, the indirect measurement of the oxygen content of arterial blood; and (5) O_2, the saturation of oxygen in the blood.

SOURCE: Klipp, 2000.

yet to be standardized and most research does not consider the total cost of an episode of care, it is difficult to compare findings that might help laboratory managers choose the most appropriate type of testing (Baer, 1998). It is also difficult to measure the convenience to patients and physicians of POCT. Some experts, however, expect the value of POCT to Medicare beneficiaries to be high, particularly in physicians' offices.

In some cases, there may be a trade-off between the convenience of POCT and quality. Steven Gutman, M.D., director of the Food and Drug Administration's (FDA's) division of clinical laboratory devices points out that POCT devices may not have to meet the same quality standards as laboratory-based testing (Uehling, 2000). Some devices, such as a video microscope used to visualize and count blood cells, may even be exempt from FDA review and subject to only minimal oversight under the Clinical Laboratory Improvement Amendments (CLIA) (Uehling, 2000). David Wilkinson, chairman of the Department of Pathology at the Medical College of Virginia, points out that some POCT systems have a high failure rate of disposable cartridges that house the analytical components, and there may be test result bias when compared to central laboratory methods (Wilkinson, 1997).

TABLE 3.2 Home Testing Market by Sector, 1999

Sector	Expenditures ($ million)
Blood glucose monitoring	1,590
Pregnancy, ovulation test kits	153
HIV sample collection kits	10
Cholesterol monitoring test kits	3
Drugs-of-abuse kits	3

SOURCE: Klipp, 2000.

Home Testing

Home testing is another growing market made possible by technological advances in laboratory testing. Unlike POCT, home testing is decentralized and physicians may not receive the test results unless they are provided manually by patients or entered into shared Internet-based data-monitoring systems. This has not limited the growth of the home testing market. In 1999, the total amount spent on home testing was $2.1 billion. Table 3.2 shows the sectors of the home testing market in 1999. These home testing products are relatively inexpensive, over-the-counter diagnostic and monitoring kits and devices.

The home test market is consumer driven. Home-based tests are purchased by consumers and are rarely covered by third-party payers. Nevertheless, the demand for these products continues to increase. The $1.7 billion market in 1997 is expected to increase 100 percent by 2004 (Klipp, 2000). Future technologies may enable patients to take a more active role in their own care, integrating home testing into their medical regime. Some experts foresee a time when patients will be able to view, interpret, and add important information to their medical records through Internet-linked, hand-held devices designed for home use. They will also be able to use diagnostic products purchased from a grocery store or pharmacy and automatically upload the results to their electronic medical records in the privacy of their homes (Felder et al., 1999). The home-based test market is unlikely to completely replace sophisticated hospital and independent laboratories, especially in light of the ever-growing number of complex tests.

EFFECT ON CLINICAL LABORATORY STAFF REQUIREMENTS

Not surprisingly, the recent and ongoing changes in clinical laboratory technology have had an impact on laboratory staff needs. According to Kenneth Cruse, MT American Society of Clinical Pathologists (ASCP), "Traditionally, nontechnical staff collected specimens from patients and gave the specimens to technicians to perform the tests" (Cruse, 1998). Nontechnical staff members still do many of the repetitive jobs, such as feeding specimen tubes onto highly automated instruments throughout the facility.[15] Technical staff members now conduct preventive maintenance on laboratory equipment, run quality control specimens, and correct identified problems. They also evaluate patient results that require a manual review (Cruse, 1998). Highly skilled laboratorians with clinical and analytical knowledge are still essential to perform and interpret many of the more sophisticated tests.

The growth in automation and robotics is decreasing the need for nontechnical staff in the laboratory (Wilkinson, 1997). Labor cost savings may be offset somewhat by a need for additional IT staff to monitor and maintain the automated systems (Sainato, 2000). Growth in point-of-care tests, which do not have to be performed by physicians, may mean that more allied health personnel will be needed in hospitals and physicians' offices.

In the future, growth in the number of esoteric tests may increase the demand for highly skilled staff. Some predict that the number of clinical laboratory technologists and technicians is not expected to keep pace with the demand for laboratory services over the next decade, especially in the areas of cytogenetics, tissue typing, genetic testing, and transplantation. Others predict that the same trends that have reduced the need for nontechnical staff will affect the need for skilled staff (Burtis, 1996; Maibach et al., 1998).

Perhaps the greatest savings in laboratory costs will come from technology that enables labor reduction (Felder et al., 1999). For example, the move to total laboratory automation could reduce labor costs by 25–50 percent (Jacobs and Simson, 1999). Reducing the need for labor could have profound effects on the cost of performing testing since labor constitutes approximately 60 percent of the total cost of laboratory services (Jacobs and Simson, 1999). Kenneth Cruse argues that other benefits of redistributing work among technical and nontechnical personnel include enhanced productivity, increased testing accuracy and precision, significant reduction of TATs, increased physician satisfaction levels, and the potential to reduce the length of stay for hospitalized patients (Cruse, 1998).

SUMMARY

Clinical laboratories are in the midst of a technological revolution that is likely to continue during the twenty-first century. Many medical advances will be led by technological innovation in laboratory testing. New technology is positively associated with increased efficiency, reduction in errors, and improved quality in the delivery of health care services. Whether new technologies

---

[15]As noted in footnote 6, when considering the tasks conducted by individuals who do not have technical skills, it is important to note that many states have licensure laws that preclude the conduct of certain testing procedures by nontechnical staff. In addition, CLIA requirements, as they relate to moderate- and high-complexity tests, do not allow the use of nontechnical staff for certain testing procedures.

are implemented may depend on their impact on laboratory costs and, if they are more costly, on payers' willingness to pay for them.

While efforts to automate central laboratories are likely to continue, trends appear to indicate that much routine testing in the future could be delivered through POCT and home-based testing. Centralized laboratories are likely to concentrate more on esoteric testing. Automation and shifts in the sites where laboratory services are delivered will result in major shifts in laboratory staffing needs. Demand for skilled IT professionals, experts to monitor and service robotic equipment, and allied health professionals is likely to grow. Overall decreases in labor costs, however, will likely lead to decreases in the cost per test.

REFERENCES

Baer, D. M. 1998. Point-of-care testing versus central lab costs. *MLO Med Lab Obs* 30, No. 9:46-56.

Berger, A., and R. Smith. 1999. Editorial: New technologies in medicine and medical journals. *BMJ* 319. Available at: http://www.bmj.com/cgi/content/full/319/7220/0.

Burtis, C. A. 1996. Converging technologies and their impact on the clinical laboratory. *Clin Chem* 42, No. 11:1735–1749.

Children's Health Care System. 1999. GeneTests. Web page, accessed July 31, 2000. Available at www.genetests.org. Funded by the National Library of Medicine, National Institutes of Health and the Maternal and Child Health Bureau, Health Resources and Services Administration.

Chou, D. 1996. Internet: Road to heaven or hell for the clinical laboratory? *Clin Chem* 42, No. 5:827–830.

Cruse, K. L. 1998. Timeliness and best demonstrated practices. *Clin Lab Manage Rev* 12, No. 3:159–168.

Direct-to-consumer test result reporting: Should it be in your lab's future? 2000. *Clinical Laboratory Strategies* 5, No. 3.

Evans, W. E., and M. V. Relling. 1999. Pharmacogenomics: Translating functional genomics into rational therapeutics. *Science* 286, No. 5439:487–491.

Executive Office of the President of the United States. 2000. The National Nanotechnology Initiative. Web page, accessed September 5, 2000. Available at www.nano.gov.

Felder, R. A., S. Graves, and T. Mifflin. 1999. Reading the future: The increased relevance of laboratory medicine in the next century. *MLO Med Lab Obs* 31, No. 7:20-21, 24–26.

Friedman, B. A. 1998. Integrating laboratory processes into clinical processes, Web-based laboratory reporting, and the emergence of the virtual clinical laboratory. *Clin Lab Manage Rev* 12, No. 5:333–338.

Holtzman, N. A. 1999. Promoting safe and effective genetic tests in the United States: Work of the task force on genetic testing. *Clin Chem* 45, No. 5:732–738.

Holtzman, N. A., and T. Marteau. 2000. Will genetics revolutionize medicine? *N Engl J Med* 343, No. 2:141–144.

Howanitz, P. 1994. From start to finish, how accurate are lab tests? *CAP Today,* pp. 41–42.

Jacobs, E., and E. Simson. December 1999. Point-of-care testing, and laboratory automation. *Clinical Laboratory News,* pp. 12–14.

Jones, S. 2000. *Genetics in Medicine: Real Promises, Unreal Expectations: One Scientist's Advice to Policymakers in the United Kingdom and the United States.* New York: Milbank Memorial Fund.

Kendall, J., B. Reeves, and M. Clancy. 1998. Point of care testing: Randomized controlled trial of clinical outcome [see comments]. *BMJ* 316, No. 7137:1052–1057. Comment in BMJ 1998; 317 No. 7161: 818–819.

Klatt, E. C. 1997. Open your laboratory to the Internet. *MLO Med Lab Obs* 29, No. 11:28–32.

Klipp, J. 2000. *Lab Industry Strategic Outlook 2000: Market Trends & Analysis.* Washington, DC: Washington G-2 Reports.

Lifshitz, M., and R. De Cresce. 1989. Automation: Trends in instrumentation, robotics, and computers. MLO *Med Lab Obs* 21, No. 7:73–77.

Maibach, H., R. Keenlyside, D. Fitzmaurice, D. Brogan, and J. Essien. 1998. Future directions for research in laboratory medicine: The findings of a Delphi survey of stakeholders. *Clin Lab Manage Rev* 12, No. 4:221–230; discussion 231.

Marietti, C. August 1998. Golden labs: Laboratories look to newer systems to streamline labor-intensive tasks, reduce payrolls and speed turnaround times. *Healthcare Informatics,* pp. 65–77.

Markin, R. S., and S. A. Whalen. 2000. Laboratory automation: trajectory, technology, and tactics. *Clin Chem* 46, No. 5:764–771.

McDonald, J. M. 1997. The value-added laboratory: An opportunity to merge research and service objectives. *Clin Lab Manage Rev* 11, No. 2:88–92.

McGee, P. 2000. Sizing Up Nanotechnology. Web page, available at www.wired.com/news/technology/0,1282,37217,00.html.

McPherson, R. A. 1998. Robotics, automation, and the new role of process control. *Clinical Laboratory Management Review,* pp. 339–346.

Nakamura, R. M. 1999. Technology that will initiate future revolutionary changes in healthcare and the clinical laboratory. *J Clin Lab Anal* 13, No. 2:49–52.

Parvin, C. A., S. F. Lo, S. M. Deuser, L. W. Weaver, L. M. Lewis, and M. G. Scott. 1996. Impact of point-of-care testing on patients' length of stay in a large emergency department. *Clinical Chemistry* 42, No. 5:711–717.

Plebani, M. 1999. The changing face of clinical laboratories. *Clin Chem Lab Med* 37, No. 7:711–717.

Roco, M. C., S. Williams, and P. Alivisatos. Applications: Biological, Medical, and Health. September 1999. *Nanotechnology Research Directions: IWGN Workshop Report: Vision for Nanotechnology Research and Development in the Next Decade.* Baltimore, MD: WTEC, Loyola College in Maryland.

Root, C. B. 1997. In Office Testing, Just What the Doctor Ordered. Barrington, IL: (unpublished).

Rose, W. D., J. E. Martin, F. M. Abraham, R. L. Jackson, J. M. Williams, and E. Gunel. 1997. Calcium, magnesium, and phosphorus: Emergency department testing yield. *Academic Emergency Medicine* 4, No. 6:559–563.

Sainato, D. April 1999. POCT vs. central lab testing. *Clinical Laboratory News,* p. 15.

Sainato, D. January 2000. Laboratory automation: Coming of age in the 21st century. *Clinical Laboratory News,* pp. 1, 6–7.

Smith Barney. 1995. *Smith Barney Draft White Paper: Overview of the Clinical Laboratory Industry.* New York, NY: Smith Barney.

Travers, E. M., and C. F. Krochmal. 1988. A new way to determine test cost per instrument. Part I. *MLO Med Lab Obs* 20, No. 10:24–29.

Tsai, W. W., D. B. Nash, B. Seamonds, and G. J. Weir. 1994. Point-of-care versus central laboratory testing: An economic analysis in an academic medical center. *Clin Ther* 16, No. 5:898–910; discussion 854.

Uehling, M. July 2000. Under the skin: Sorting through the hype and hope for noninvasive POC devices. *CAP Today,* pp. 52, 56, 62, 66, 68.

Van Heyningen, C., I. D. Watson, and A. E. Morrice. 1999. Point-of-care testing outcomes in an emergency department. *Clinical Chemistry* , 45 No. 3:437–438.

Weiss, R. 24 June 2000. The promise of precision prescriptions. *Washington Post,* section A, pp. 1,16.

Where is the lab industry headed in the next decade? February 2000. *Clinical Laboratory News,* p. 12.

Wilkinson, D. S. 1997. The role of technology in the clinical laboratory of the future. *Clin Lab Manage Rev* 11, No. 5:322–330.

Woo, J., and J. B. Henry. 1994. The advance of technology as a prelude to the laboratory of the twenty-first century. *Clin Lab Med* 14, No. 3:459–471.

4
Description of the Current Medicare Payment System and Its Historical Roots

Medicare currently pays for outpatient clinical laboratory tests according to a prospective system using a specific payment for each test or service, set separately in fee schedules for each of 56 geographic jurisdictions, and limited by a national cap. The current system has evolved over almost two decades, with many changes resulting from either legislative mandates or administrative decisions. It is an extremely complex system with no clear map to guide a newcomer. Hence the committee devoted considerable effort to collecting official documents and data and talking with experts from all aspects of the payment system.

INTRODUCTION

This chapter provides a guide to the current payment methodology and its historical roots, as well as a foundation for further analytical work in later chapters. Because payment policy for laboratory services is so deeply entwined with other policy issues such as how new tests are approved for marketing, assigned billing codes and Medicare coverage, and how claims are processed, the committee found that changes are needed in these areas to support the recommendations it makes about payment policy. To provide context for these recommendations, these issues are briefly reviewed. The final section of this chapter focuses on payment policy. It begins with a brief history of payment policy prior to the development of the current payment system, discusses how the current system evolved, and ends with a discussion of elements of the current payment system. These elements are used as a framework in Chapter 6 when payment alternatives are considered.

Much of the research for this chapter is based on evidence provided by testimony to the committee, interviews and discussions with many individuals within the Health Care Financing Administration (HCFA), Medicare contractors, other federal regulators, and numerous members of the laboratory industry and their associations. In addition, it relies on reports and data from the committee's consultants, the General Accounting Office (GAO), the Office of the Inspector General (OIG) of the Department of Health and Human Services (DHHS), and the Clinical Laboratory Improvement Act (CLIA) program.

THE FDA APPROVAL PROCESS

Before Medicare considers a new technology, the new test or technology must be reviewed by the Food and Drug Administration (FDA) to determine whether it is safe and effective. The FDA approval process does not consider costs, impact on disease treatment, or patient outcomes. In granting approval, the FDA is simply approving marketing. No representation is made to Medicare or any other insurer about whether the test is worth covering in its benefit package or how it should be used.

Of the approximately 1,000 new clinical laboratory tests and technologies that come to the FDA for review annually, about 99 percent are considered substantially equivalent to existing tests (Silva, 2000). These receive an abbreviated review called a 510K Pre-Market Notification and are approved if their performance is approximately 90–95 percent the same as that of the existing, comparable test (Medical Device Act). The few new tests that are significantly different from existing tests go through a more extensive Pre-Market Approval (PMA) process. For a PMA, the manufacturer must prove, through clinical studies, that the new test or technology is safe and effective.

CODING POLICY

Laboratory services are billed using the HCFA Common Procedural Coding System (HCPCS). HCPCS codes include the physicians' Current Procedural Terminology (CPT) codes, which are controlled and published by the American Medical Association (AMA), plus local and national temporary codes assigned by contractors and HCFA. Some of these codes are used for billing other payers besides Medicare.

Coding Updates

Each year, CPT code changes include the addition of new tests, new panels, or changes in the composition of panels including tests previously coded individually. HCFA receives the AMA's CPT changes in July, although some are known months earlier. HCFA physicians and other staff review the code changes during the summer and begin "mapping" the changes, based on guidance from the AMA. That is, they translate the location of an existing test (and its related code) in the previous coding system to its location in the updated codes, so that the previous fees can be attached to the new code. All changes have to be resolved by the end of October because the new fee schedule goes to the contractors on November 1 to allow them time to implement the changes before fees take effect at the start of the next calendar year.

Panel Codes

The AMA's CPT Editorial Panel groups certain tests together for the convenience of physicians and claims processors. It has changed the composition of various panels several times since the mid-1980s, requiring corresponding changes in the payment system. For example, some time ago, the composition of multichannel test panels was changed to permit the inclusion of unrelated tests. This created problems because physicians were not aware that possibly unrelated and unnecessary tests were included in the panel and that those tests were billed separately to Medicare in addition to the standard panel of tests intentionally ordered. This opportunity for fraud and abuse was targeted by the Inspector General and the panels were redefined. The OIG also raised concerns about the medical necessity of all the tests billed in large panels and, in other cases, questioned the laboratories' unbundling of panel tests to maximize payments by billing for each test individually. Now, panels include tests that either are all related to the analysis of a specific organ's functions, are standard for the diagnosis of particular diseases, or are commonly ordered together for multiple diagnostic purposes. Nonetheless, the physician and the laboratory must not bill for an entire panel code unless the patient needs each test. If the full panel is not needed, the tests can be ordered individually.

Codes for New Technology

If a new test is similar in method or analyte (the substance being measured) to an existing test or combination of tests, it may be assigned the same code. At other times, a new test may be assigned a new code, but the payment amount for that code may be linked to an existing code or combination of codes. Tests that receive 510K approval from the FDA are more likely to be assigned an existing code.

If a manufacturer believes a new test is significantly different from existing technology or has a significantly different cost than current payment rates for existing codes, the manufacturer is free to request a new code for the test from the AMA's CPT Editorial Panel. Seeking a new code can be a time-consuming process and may slow the introduction of new technology.

Alternatively, manufacturers may choose to disseminate new technology without a new CPT code, leaving laboratories to use a miscellaneous "catch-all" CPT code for billing purposes. Occasionally contractors or HCFA assign a local or temporary HCPCS code for billing purposes. Some initially temporary codes, such as the code for venipuncture, have become permanent.

Ambiguities in Code Use

Although in concept there is a separate code for each service, in practice it does not always happen this way. Some codes refer to the analyte, such as a tumor antigen marker in blood, and may encompass several different measurement methods. Other codes identify a particular testing methodology, such as a generic immunoassay or generic tumor marker, rather than what is being measured. Thus, a single CPT code may identify more than one testing method for a given substance or more than one analyte measured by a single method.

With more than 1,100 distinct codes, it is not always clear to a physician or laboratory how to identify a particular service, especially if it is new. In these situations, the CPT decision hierarchy indicates that (1) coding by analyte is the preferred choice, then (2) coding by methodology, and finally (3) the "99" code for "miscellaneous" is the last option. Some carriers either routinely deny claims from the miscellaneous category or set the payment rate for that code at $0.00.

The ambiguities of the coding system create a challenge for any payment methodology. If there is uncertainty about exactly what is included under a particular code, it is difficult to know whether the fee or payment is appropriate. For some services, "apples and oranges" are combined under the same code, and the fee may be appropriate for the apple, but not for the orange. For example, if both available testing methods produce the same result in the same time frame, but vary substantially in cost, it is not a concern for Medicare as long as the fee reflects the less expensive version. The coding issue becomes more problematic when a new version of a test may produce a better-quality result or a faster turnaround time but costs substantially more than the payment amount linked to the code.

CLAIMS PROCESSING

Medicare contractors play a variety of important roles. They are the key link between the policymakers in HCFA headquarters and the laboratory providers. Their basic function is to receive and process claims and make payments. There are approximately 53 different contractors, some with multiple contracts, covering all of the 56 jurisdictions. The fiscal intermediaries (FIs), contractors for hospital-based laboratories, or the carriers, contractors for physician office laboratories (POLs) and independent laboratories, handle daily program operations. Because of their numbers and separate jurisdictions, their operations vary. This can cause problems for laboratories, primarily large independent and referral laboratories, that deal with specimens from many states.

Based on industry urging, Congress included language in the 1997 Balanced Budget Act (BBA) requiring HCFA to consolidate its contractor functions for laboratories into four or five regional laboratory carriers (RLCs). One of the

RLCs is to be designated the Central Statistical Carrier (CSC) with added responsibility to provide analyses of laboratory claims and utilization issues. HCFA is now implementing this provision. The administration originally opposed the provision, in part because of the substantial additional expense to convert and operate the RLCs for the first five years.

HCFA plans to have the regional laboratory carriers fully functioning within two years of resolving policy and operational issues. HCFA consolidated carriers for durable medical equipment (DME) suppliers in 1993, and they appear to be running smoothly, but there has not yet been an evaluation of the changes. HCFA reports that the DME consolidation has promoted greater consistency in program operations and led to better control of fraud and abuse.

It is too soon to predict how the RLC consolidation will affect the clinical laboratory payment system. The success of this effort will depend on many policy decisions yet to be made, including the following:

- Will any categories of laboratory claims be excluded from the consolidation? Will hospital-based laboratories continue to bill the hospital's fiscal intermediary? Will POLs continue to bill the physician's carrier?
- Should local coverage policy remain or become consolidated at the regional level? What will the process be for creating future medical review policies?
- What entities should become RLCs and how will they be selected?
- How will regional claims data be consolidated to provide a stronger capability for detecting patterns of fraud and abuse?
- How will consolidation affect payment levels in different states?

The way this consolidation proceeds, and how fast it occurs will have significant implications for the current payment methodology and any changes to be made to it. The committee anticipated this consolidation when it made its recommendations. Ideally, implementation of the recommendations in Chapter 7 should be planned in conjunction with plans for the RLCs. Many of the policy issues are interdependent, and the changes have to be coordinated carefully to avoid overloading the computer systems and all the stakeholders.

MEDICARE COVERAGE POLICY

Coverage policy is separate and distinct from payment policy, but directly affects the operation of the payment system.[1] Payment for a particular service depends on Medicare recognition that the service is covered—that it is within the legislative mandate to provide medically necessary diagnostic and treatment services. Medicare specifically excludes some categories of health care, such as

---

[1]"A Medicare coverage decision, whether made nationally or locally, is a prospective, population-based, policy that applies to a clinical subset or class of Medicare beneficiaries and describes the clinical circumstances and setting under which an item or service is available (or is not available)" (Medicare Program, 2000).

most preventive and screening services and most treatments that have not obtained FDA approval. Coverage decisions affect whether and how quickly new technologies are incorporated into the payment system. About 10 percent of new Medicare items and services receive coverage decisions at the national level; the remaining 90 percent are handled locally by HCFA's contractors.

Without coding and coverage decisions at the national level, contractors usually determine coverage policy for laboratory services. Frequently, a manufacturer markets a new test selectively in certain geographic areas. The carrier in these areas may require documentation of medical necessity and appropriateness along with the claims from the physician and the laboratory, and may also make case-by-case determinations of whether the test is covered.

National Coverage Decisions

As use of a new test increases and more carriers make decisions about coverage and payment, the coverage issue may rise to the national level at HCFA. A CPT code assignment by the AMA may also make the coverage issue more visible at the national level. Alternatively, the manufacturer and interested clinicians may request HCFA to make a national coverage decision, which is binding on all contractors. This is often difficult since experience with the new technology is required, and to collect that experience, laboratories have to be paid for conducting the test.

New, more clear, open, and speedy national coverage procedures were announced in 1999 (Medicare Program, 1999), which should facilitate national coverage decisions at HCFA. Still, it may take from six months to several years for a new test to be approved nationally for coverage (Lewin Group, 2000). For complex, new technologies, HCFA will seek the advice of its Medicare Coverage Advisory Committee (MCAC), which has a Clinical Laboratory Subcommittee. This step could add to the processing time required. The MCAC will offer recommendations to HCFA based on literature reviews, technology assessment data, and expert advice.

Criteria for evaluating new tests and procedures include consideration of scientific evidence concerning patient outcomes, although such data are rare. In the past, costs were not considered in the Medicare coverage policy decision, although this has been a controversial topic of debate. In May 2000, HCFA issued a notice of intent to publish new review criteria that include a cost consideration when the new service offers substantially the same benefit as a currently covered service (Medicare Program, 2000). The proposed criteria allow coverage if the new service results in equivalent or lower costs for the same Medicare populations than the Medicare-covered alternative. New services that provide more benefits than currently approved services will be covered, regardless of costs.

Local Medical Review Policy

Carriers and FIs process claims and determine whether services being billed are medically necessary. This is an important function, since Medicare pays only for covered services that are medically necessary in each particular case. Because contractors process billions of claims annually, computers make most of the determinations, based on data submitted on the claim. To facilitate the decision process, carriers use local carrier advisory committees (CACs) to develop local medical review policies (LMRPs) for new tests and for tests that are overused. There may be laboratory representation on the CAC, but the local laboratory industry and manufacturers generally do not have direct input into the decision process and learn about new coverage issues only after the carrier makes a decision and notifies providers. The LMRPs state which conditions and diagnoses the contractor considers appropriate (or inappropriate) for a given test. The FIs generally, but not always, follow the LMRPs of the local carrier.

Because each carrier develops its LMRPs independently, there is considerable variation among the LMRPs concerning which tests need a policy at all and which of the International Classification of Diseases, Ninth Revision, (ICD-9) diagnosis and symptom codes are acceptable to justify the medical necessity of the test. Laboratories that test specimens from different geographic jurisdictions must be familiar with the carriers' LMRPs in each jurisdiction in order to file claims properly. This is a challenge for large national and reference laboratories.

LMRPs require that claims for certain tests include an ICD-9 diagnosis code. Laboratories bill Medicare directly, so they must rely on physicians to provide these diagnosis codes when they order tests. Physicians may have difficulty identifying an appropriate diagnosis code, since the test may be used to make the diagnosis. However, some ICD-9 codes indicate a range of symptoms and are used when no diagnosis is available. Physicians may be reluctant to share diagnostic information with the laboratory because of concerns about patient confidentiality. Laboratorians feel an obligation to the patient and often conduct the test even though they do not have adequate information to bill Medicare for the test. Laboratory personnel spend a considerable amount of time calling physicians to collect diagnostic information required for Medicare billing.

Coverage determinations for new laboratory tests are a potpourri of statutory constraints, national coverage determinations, and local carrier decision making. Although coverage determinations, particularly at the national level, may be time consuming, the committee found no systematic evidence to suggest clinically important delays in Medicare beneficiaries' access to new clinical laboratory technologies.

Claims Denials

Claims for tests are denied when they (1) are for tests not covered by Medicare; (2) do not satisfy medical necessity requirements as defined by Medicare; (3) are for persons who are not Medicare beneficiaries; (4) are from laboratories that are not Medicare providers or not CLIA-certified to perform the particular test; (5) are insufficiently documented; or (6) are for patients who have primary coverage from another payer. Claims denials are important because they affect the cost of providing laboratory services. Even if payments cover the costs of individual tests, they will not compensate for claims denials, which increase administrative costs, reduce the aggregate Medicare revenue for laboratories, and create bad debt.

Medicare's national claims denial rates for the top 100 laboratory tests in terms of dollar volume ranged from 6 to 39 percent, according to 1998 HCFA claims data (Appendix E). Although all third-party payers deny claims on occasion, testimony from those in the laboratory industry indicates a perception that Medicare denial rates greatly exceed those of other third parties. No evidence was available to support or refute this impression. The committee's examination of Medicare's denial rates showed that 26 CPT codes out of 100 had denial rates of 20 percent or more. Only 25 of the top 100 tests had denial rates that were not in the double digits (Appendix E). The overall denial rate for the 100 highest-volume test codes for outpatient laboratory claims processed by carriers nationally was 15 percent in 1998. (Claims data from the FIs for hospital-based laboratories were unavailable.)

These data are confounded by the fact that denied claims can be resubmitted and appealed. Although the number of claims ultimately denied is no doubt lower than the number initially denied, there is no information available regarding the size of this differential.

For the top 20 laboratory tests (by dollar volume) by carrier, denial rates varied substantially by region. For example, the lipoprotein assay (CPT-83718) was denied 68 percent of the time in Montana, 48 percent in Alabama, and only 7 percent in Washington. Some potential explanations for this variation include (1) geographic patterns of fraud and abuse, (2) interpretation of Medicare rules by local carriers, and (3) low numbers of tests in a region that easily skew the proportion of denied claims.

Information explaining reasons for the denials is not available.[2] The committee does not know the percentage of claims denied on grounds of medical necessity, that is, claims that contain inappropriate diagnosis codes or are missing diagnostic information. However, laboratorians suggest that medical necessity is the primary reason for denials. Information was not available on how much medical necessity denial rates vary by carrier. Some potential causes of variation are unusually restrictive LMRPs in some areas and differences in interpretation of national coverage rules by local carriers. It is unclear how many of the denials result from coding errors, incomplete documentation, confusion over coverage policies, and inappropriate utilization (as defined by local or national medical review policies).

[2]The committee did learn from HCFA that 2.5 percent of claims submitted by POLs were denied based on a lack of medical necessity.

When a claim is denied on grounds of medical necessity, the laboratory generally bears the financial burden. The laboratory can attempt to collect additional data from the physician to justify medical necessity and then resubmit the claim. If this fails, the laboratory can attempt to collect from the beneficiary; however, beneficiaries can be billed only if they were warned, prior to receiving the test, that it might not be covered. Alternatively, the laboratory can attempt to collect from the physician, but it appears that most laboratories are reluctant to bill physicians since they are considered the laboratory's prime customers.

Advanced Beneficiary Notice

When physicians have reason to think Medicare might consider a test medically inappropriate in a particular case, they are obliged to advise the beneficiary of this possibility and have the patient sign an Advanced Beneficiary Notice (ABN) acknowledging the warning and accepting responsibility to pay for the test. In those situations, the laboratory is allowed to bill the beneficiary if Medicare denies the claim. Since the laboratory rarely has direct contact with the beneficiary, it depends on the physicians to recognize that the ordered test is subject to a medical review policy, to acknowledge that medical necessity is not obvious, and to obtain a signature on an ABN from the patient. Although this sounds straightforward, there are many nuances that can affect the use of ABNs.

When a national laboratory association attempted to clarify the language and use of ABNs under particular circumstances, an extended correspondence with HCFA ensued. HCFA's responses set important policies for the program, but they have never been communicated publicly to all contractors and providers, so substantial variations in practice continue. For example, in 1996, HCFA approved the use of ABNs for screening tests such as the Pap test that have statutorily mandated frequency limits. HCFA encouraged specifically worded ABN forms to be used, depending on particular circumstances, but it has yet to promulgate the forms and instructions for their use. In addition, since it is impossible for the physician or laboratory to know whether the patient has already received the screening test within the defined period of time, the provider has no way of knowing which version of the ABN is appropriate. Another complication is the legal ambiguity of physicians billing patients.

Negotiated Rulemaking

In an attempt to rationalize some of the variations in LMRPs, in 1998–1999 HCFA conducted a negotiated rulemaking, as directed by the 1997 Balanced Budget Act.[3] The appointed committee developed national coverage policies for

---

[3]In a negotiated rulemaking process, a committee of representatives of stakeholders that may be affected by the rule, including agency representatives, is formed with the aim of reaching consensus on the content and text of a proposed rule. Specific procedures are followed to ensure an impartial process.

23 different tests, including many of the most commonly conducted tests. HCFA estimates that the 23 national coverage policies would cover 60 percent of the dollar volume of outpatient claims. These and other national coverage policies take precedence over LMRPs. The resulting proposed rule, referred to as the Neg Reg and published in March 2000, will not take full effect until one year after the final rule is published (HCFA, 2000a). The hope is that it will improve the consistency of claims processing and medical necessity determinations.

Coverage policies specify the appropriate ICD-9 codes for certain tests. After implementation of the Neg Reg, if the physician fails to include a required ICD-9 code, the contractor will attempt to obtain this information (HCFA, 2000a). It currently is the responsibility of the laboratory to request the documentation from the physician. This will relieve the laboratories of an administrative burden, but will not eliminate their ultimate responsibility for the bill if the physician cannot or will not document the claim appropriately and the laboratory is reluctant to bill the physician.

MEDICARE PAYMENT POLICY

Early History of the Payment System

The current payment system dates from changes initiated in 1984. Prior to that time, covered laboratory services ordered by a physician and performed in the physician's office or in an independent laboratory were paid by Part B on a "reasonable charge" basis. Medicare payments to these laboratories were based on charges, not costs.[4] Four primary calculations were used to determine the reasonable charge; the lowest of these four calculations was the "reasonable charge":

1. **Actual charge:** This is actual charge billed for service by a physician or an independent laboratory.
2. **Customary charge:** This represents the physician's or the laboratory's customary charge for the service, equal to the median charge for that particular service for the past year.
3. **Prevailing charge:** Within a locality, this represents the 75th percentile of all customary charges for the test, weighted by volume.
4. **Lowest charge:** Some common laboratory tests were designated as tests that do not vary significantly in quality among providers. These were reimbursed at the 25th percentile of the full array of actual charges billed to the carrier within a locality during a given period.

When an independent laboratory performed a test on a sample submitted by a physician, the physician would pay the laboratory for the test, often at a dis-

---

[4]Payments to hospitals for outpatient tests were based on costs, as were other hospital services.

counted rate. The physician would then bill Medicare for the service. The "reasonable charge" of the independent laboratory was used as the basis for Medicare payment to the physician. The Omnibus Budget Reconciliation Act of 1980 (OBRA 1980) stipulated that if the physician did not identify the laboratory or the amount charged him, payment would be based on the lowest amount at which the test could have been obtained from a laboratory in the area. For tests other than those performed in the physician's own laboratory, the physician was permitted to charge a separate fee for drawing, collecting, or handling a specimen, not to exceed $3.00 in most cases.

Payment under Part B for laboratory services performed in a POL or in an independent laboratory, where the laboratory collected the sample, was made either directly to the patient or, in the case of assignment, to the independent laboratory or the physician. Assignment meant that the laboratory or physician billed Medicare directly and was paid directly on the basis of 80 percent of the reasonable charge for the service minus any outstanding deductible amount. The laboratory or physician could then charge the beneficiary no more than 20 percent of the reasonable charge (coinsurance), plus the portion of the deductible not yet paid by the beneficiary. In the case of an unassigned claim, the beneficiary filed a claim with Medicare, and Medicare paid 80 percent of the reasonable charge minus any outstanding deductible amount. The independent laboratory or POL billed the beneficiary, and the beneficiary was responsible for paying the laboratory including any charges in excess of what Medicare computed as "reasonable."

DEVELOPMENT OF THE CURRENT SYSTEM

The Deficit Reduction Act of 1984 (DEFRA) introduced radical changes to the payment methodology for Medicare Part B clinical laboratory services, including (1) establishment of area-wide fee schedules, (2) direct billing by the provider that performed the test, and (3) elimination of the beneficiary copayments for services to be billed on an assigned basis (Logue, 1996). Under DEFRA, Congress established prospectively set carrier fee schedules for laboratories (Section 1833(h) of the Social Security Act). The fee schedules were based on prevailing charges, which in turn were based on 1983 customary charge data. The 75th percentile of customary charges defined the prevailing charge in a given area. There was a mechanism to update fees annually, based on the change in the Consumer Price Index (CPI). For most years, however, Congress has specified lower update factors (Table 4.1). The fee schedules varied by local carrier area. The intent was to move toward a national fee schedule. However, in 1987 OBRA 1987 postponed this requirement, and in 1989 it was completely repealed.

Effective July 1, 1984, laboratories were paid based on the lower of submitted charges or the fee schedule rate. For hospital-based laboratories (outpa-

TABLE 4.1 Medicare Laboratory Fee Schedule Updates and National Limitation Amount Percentages, 1984–2002

Year	Fee Schedule Update (%)	Percentage of Median Used to Set NLA
1984	CPI-U	NA
1985	CPI-U	NA
1986	CPI-U	115
1987	CPI-U	115
1988	0.0	100
1989	4.0	100
1990	CPI-U	93
1991	2.0	88
1992	2.0	88
1993	2.0	88
1994	0.0	84
1995	0.0	80
1996	2.9	76
1997	2.7	76
1998–2002	0.0	74

NOTE: CPI-U = Consumer Price Index-Urban, published by the U.S. Bureau of Labor Statistics; NLA = National Limitation Amount.

SOURCE: Committee on Ways and Means, 1990, 1994, 1996, and 1998.

tient services only), the fee schedule rate was set at 62 percent of the prevailing charges; for independent laboratories and POLs, the fee schedule rate was set at 60 percent of prevailing charges. The rationale for the fee reductions was evidence from several studies that laboratories were accepting fees from other payers that were significantly below the Medicare rate. These fees would be payment in full since the labs were required to accept assignment, but they were relieved of the administrative burden and bad debts associated with billing beneficiaries for a copayment.

The 1985 Consolidated Omnibus Budget Reconciliation Act (COBRA) mandated that HCFA impose National Limitation Amounts (NLAs) for clinical laboratory fees beginning in July 1986. The NLAs were set at 115 percent of the median of all local fee schedule amounts for each procedure. Reflecting congressional budget actions over the years, HCFA has substantially decreased the level of the NLAs. In 1999, the NLAs were set at 74 percent of the median.

ELEMENTS OF A PAYMENT SYSTEM

Establishing the amount that a health service provider is paid for providing services to patients involves decisions in several different dimensions.[5,6] This section first lists the various elements of a payment system, then continues with a discussion of the current laboratory payment methodology. Decisions about the nature of these payment elements for any payment approach must answer the following questions:

- Do the provider, patient, and payer all know what the payment amount is when a service is provided?
- What is the payment for?
- What is payment based on?
- What determines the payment level?
- How do payments change over time?
- Are payments adjusted for any specific provider or patient characteristics or circumstances?
- How much does the patient pay?

The answers to these questions determine the financial incentives that affect how health services are produced and consumed.

An additional factor complicating the incentive structure for laboratory services is the fact that patients use services based on a referral from their physician. The laboratory has three different customers: the patient, the ordering physician, and the third-party payer. The tension between these three creates unusual incentives.

This section describes the seven basic elements of a payment system that respond to the questions above, including (1) type of payment, (2) unit of payment, (3) basis of payment, (4) level of payment, (5) payment updates, (6) adjustments, and (7) cost sharing.

Type of Payment

Payments are either *retrospective* or *prospective*. In a retrospective system, the actual payment amount at the time of the service is unknown to at least some of the actors. In prospective systems, providers, payers and patients are able to know how much the laboratory will be paid for a test before the test is ordered or the service provided. Medicare and other payers have been moving more toward prospective payment systems.

---

[5]Much of the discussion on elements of a payment system is drawn from a paper by Katie Merrell, Center for Health Administration Studies, University of Chicago, commissioned by the Institute of Medicine (Merrell, 2000).

[6]The framework described here builds from that described by the Medicare Payment Advisory Commission (1998).

The current Medicare payment methodology for laboratory services is prospective. The fee schedule is published prior to the beginning of each calendar year for which the new fees will apply. Both HCFA and the laboratories know the price that will be paid for each test before any services are delivered.

Unit of Payment

The unit of payment describes what the payment is actually for. Payments may be for a single service, a bundled group of services, or all of the services required over a certain period of time. For example, the main difference between fee-for-service payment and capitation is the underlying unit of payment. Under fee-for-service arrangements, payment is made for each separate service (or group of services) provided, while capitated payments are made to cover a package of benefits for the covered individuals for a period of time, regardless of how many services are provided.

Examples of fee-for-service payments include a single fee for a single doctor's visit, one fee for a surgery that includes all of the preoperative and postoperative care associated with the surgical procedure, and a prenatal–delivery fee that bundles all of the visits that occur during a pregnancy. When services are bundled together, typically the payer pays less than the sum of the payments for each separate service. This creates incentives for providers to decouple the services if possible and provide them at different times, creating additional costs for the payer and inconvenience for patients. Bundling is therefore more widespread for services that cannot be divided in this way (PPRC, 1993).

Capitated payments include a monthly payment to a physician based on the number of patients assigned to his care that month or a payment to a laboratory to handle all laboratory needs for a number of patients for a specific period of time.

A provider could receive both a capitated payment to cover a selected list of common services for a given time frame and insured population and fee-for-service payments for additional, less common services needed by the same population. Some managed care organizations use this type of arrangement for purchasing laboratory services.

Under the Medicare outpatient clinical laboratory benefit, laboratory services are paid *per service or test* or per group of tests (panel). How the test is identified or coded becomes an important payment issue because the code defines what the payment covers for a specific test or service.

Basis of Payment

Payment can be based on provider charges, a fee schedule, or some negotiated amount. In some cases, there is a mixed base, with payments determined by a fee schedule to some upper limit or a combination of a fee schedule amount and actual charges. Underlying many prospective payment approaches is a basis of relative, rather than nominal, payment. In other words, the payment for a particular service is based on how it relates to the payments for other services, rather than on a specific dollar amount. The relative relationship or relative value scale (RVS)[7] can be determined in different ways—for example, by the relative relationship among charges, by negotiations, or by the resources needed to produce the various services. The current Medicare Fee Schedule for physicians reflects a resource-based relative value scale (RBRVS).[8]

Current laboratory payments are based on the 56 separate carrier fee schedule amounts, and the upper level of payment for each test is limited by an NLA.

Level of Payment

The level of payment simply refers to the actual dollar per unit of service. If the basis of payment generates dollar amounts, such as charges or a monthly capitation payment, then no separate decision is necessary to set the level of payment. In cases where the basis of payment reflects relative, rather than nominal, payment, a conversion factor is necessary to establish dollar amounts.[9] A conversion factor could be used to set the payments to accommodate a specified rate of increase or decrease in spending. For example, some payers may negotiate a discounted rate that lowers actual payment levels.

As the Medicare laboratory payment methodology has evolved, the level of payment and the formulas for setting it have changed; however, the level of payments today is closely related to the system's historical roots. Prior to the establishment of the fee schedule, Medicare payments were based on the lower of the laboratory's usual charges or the area's prevailing charges. Little is known about the relationship between the 1983 charges and the actual costs of performing the services at the time.

When Congress converted Medicare payment for laboratory services to a fee schedule in 1984, fee levels were set at 62 percent of the prevailing charge, and tests done in independent or physician office laboratories were set at 60 percent of the prevailing charge in each carrier area. In 1987, fees for outpatient services in hospital laboratories were reduced to 60 percent of the prevailing

---

[7]An RVS is an index that assigns weights to each medical service; the weights represent the relative amount to be paid for each service.

[8]In the case of the Medicare Fee Schedule for physician services, payment rates are designed to reflect relative resource use, based on separate measures of how much of a physician's work, practice expenses, and malpractice expenses each service requires relative to other services. The RBRVS is then multiplied by a conversion factor to calculate actual dollar payment amounts (PPRC, 1997).

[9]A conversion factor is used to translate the relative values for Medicare's physician fee schedule into payment amounts. The initial conversion factor was set at a level expected to maintain aggregate Medicare physician payments at the same level physicians would have received under the prior system. In other words, the conversion factor was set to maintain budget neutrality (PPRC, 1992).

charge, except for sole community provider hospitals offering 24-hour emergency room services, which remained at 62 percent.

In 1986, Congress established the National Limitation Amounts (NLAs) to serve as a ceiling on payments for each test. The NLAs are based on the median of all the carrier fees for each test. Medicare now pays the lower of the carrier's fee, the provider's charge, or the NLA. Currently, providers rarely, if ever, charge less than the carrier's fee, and the carrier's fee is usually higher that the NLA. In those cases where the NLA limits the local fee, the NLA becomes the "pricing amount"; otherwise, the pricing amount is the carrier's fee.

By the mid-1990s HCFA became aware of significant discrepancies between carrier-calculated fees and calculations made from its working files. After 1993, HCFA decided to calculate all future carrier fee schedule updates nationally along with the NLAs and to hand them back to the carriers each year. In addition, HCFA staff did a thorough reconciliation of the carriers' fees database to ensure that all previous coding changes as well as updates were accurately reflected. HCFA worked closely with the carriers to ensure a sound database and consistency for future years. The 1994 database is maintained centrally at HCFA and serves as the base year from which HCFA calculates each subsequent year's 56-carrier-area fee schedules and the NLAs.

The NLAs have been reduced repeatedly. Congress takes up Medicare policy through the budget reconciliation process and uses that process to implement cost constraints as well as policy changes in payment methods. Through the congressional budget reconciliation process, the NLAs were initially set, in 1986, at 115 percent of the median of all carriers' fees. Congress has gradually reduced the NLAs. They are now set at 74 percent of the median of the carrier fees. (Balanced Budget Act 1997, Section 4553(b)) (Table 4.1).

Because so many of the carrier fees are constrained by the NLAs, in practical terms there is now a de facto single fee schedule. Based on the calendar year (CY) 2000 fee schedule, about 85 percent of all pricing amounts (across 56 carriers and 1,100+ different test codes) were at the NLAs. Because many of the fees that are below the NLAs are in carrier jurisdictions with relatively few beneficiaries and many of the test codes with pricing amounts below the NLAs are infrequently used tests, the NLAs actually constrain spending on much more than 85 percent of the claims and much more than 85 percent of the dollar volume. According to one model (Appendix B), it appears that as much as 98 percent of all Medicare dollars paid for outpatient laboratory services are paid at the NLAs. In other words, NLAs may be the pricing amounts for more than 98 percent of laboratory claims' dollars; the NLAs appear to constrain more than 98 percent of Medicare's laboratory spending. [10]

---

[10]See Appendix B for an explanation of a commissioned study by Katie Merrell to assess the impact of the NLAs on carriers' fees. To estimate the impact of the NLA based on the volume of particular services used and the dollars paid by Medicare, it was necessary to construct a model because of data constraints. The model uses data on the number

Panel Tests

The payment level for panel tests is set differently from that for all other tests. In fact, there are currently two different types of panels, and each has payment levels set according to different formulas. There are 22 automated, multichannel chemistries such as cholesterol, calcium, glucose, potassium, uric acid, and phosphorus, which are now ordered individually but are priced according to the number of the tests ordered on the specimen, regardless of which specific tests are ordered and whether they are ordered as a full panel or individually. The theory is that the marginal costs of additional tests should be less than the cost of the first test since the specimen does not have to be logged in, processed, or handled after the first test, and all tests can be programmed into the machine once and results reported at one time. Because of historical anomalies related to the earlier grouping of more than one test into a single CPT code, the increase in payment does not relate in a consistent way to the number of tests included in the panel. In fact, there is no fee increase between panels of 12 tests and 15 tests (Table 4.2).

Other panels consist of tests that relate to a specific disease or organ function, such as the hepatic function panel. Payments for these panels are equal to the sum of the pricing amounts for the constituent tests in each carrier jurisdiction. Because the individual test pricing amounts are already limited by the NLAs, HCFA does not follow the standard test formula and select the median of the sums from all 56 carriers and reduce it by 26 percent; therefore, there are no NLAs designated for these panels.

Congressionally Set Test Payment Levels

Although Congress' main concern with the appropriateness of the level of allowed laboratory payments has been exhibited through reductions in the NLAs (changing the percentage of the median of carrier fees to be used as a cap) and constraints on inflation increases, it has also made changes in specific test fees. In 1988, Congress made a technical correction, reducing payments by 8.3 percent for certain commonly performed tests and automated chemistries. More recently, Congress addressed concerns about inadequate access to Pap smears by increasing the minimum payment. In the 1999 Balanced Budget Reconciliation Act (BBRA), Congress doubled the minimum payment for Pap tests.[11] It added, "It is the sense of the Congress that (1) the Health Care Financing Administration has been slow to incorporate or provide incentives for providers to use new screening diagnostic health care technologies in the area of cervical cancer; . . . and that the Health Care Financing Administration should institute an appropri-

---

of claims paid per test code for 85 of the 100 highest dollar volume tests, the number of beneficiaries in each of the carrier areas, and the fees for each laboratory code.

[11]Raising the price from $7.15 to $14.60.

TABLE 4.2 Panel Tests: Automated Chemistries

Number of Tests	NLA (dollars)	Marginal Increase (dollars)
2	7.20	N/A
3	9.18	1.98
4	9.69	0.51
5	10.81	1.12
6	10.84	0.03
7	11.29	0.45
8	11.70	0.41
9	12.00	0.30
10	12.00	0.00
11	12.21	0.21
12	12.48	0.27
13	12.48	0.00
14	12.48	0.00
15	12.48	0.00
16	14.61	2.13
17	14.61	0.00
18	14.71	0.10
19	15.28	0.57
20	15.78	0.50
21	16.27	0.49
22	16.77	0.50

SOURCE: HCFA, 2000b.

ate increase in the payment rate for new cervical cancer screening technologies approved by the Food and Drug Administration" (Congressional Record, H12512, Public Law 106-113, Section 224).

In addition to raising payment levels for specific tests, Congress can also reduce them. The administration's original FY 2001 budget included a proposal to reduce, by 30 percent, the NLAs for four very high volume tests that HCFA believes are currently overpaid: (1) hemoglobin (copper sulfate method, nonautomated, glycated), CPT-83036; (2) prostate-specific antigen (PSA), CPT-84153; (3) thyroid stimulating hormone (TSH), CPT-84443; and (4) urine culture (bacterial, quantitative, colony count), CPT- 87086.

Fee Level for New Technology

HCFA has established two different procedures to set the fees for new tests called ***cross-walking*** and ***gap-filling.*** Cross-walking is designed for new tests that are similar to existing tests, and gap-filling is designed for breakthrough technology. The choice of which procedure to follow depends largely on how the new technology is handled by the AMA's CPT Editorial Panel.

When a new technology is assigned an existing code, the payment amount that is attached to that code will apply to the new technology. Alternatively, if HCFA determines that the new technology is similar to two existing codes, it may combine the existing payment amounts for those codes and apply it to the new test.

The determination of which new tests can be cross-walked to which existing codes and related prices is made internally by HCFA, based on AMA advice, as it develops the next year's fee schedule. There are no published criteria guiding this process, no public description of the process, and generally no participation by stakeholders or the public. There is no official process for stakeholders to challenge these decisions.

When a testing product is so new that there is little upon which to base payment, the payment amount for the product is gap-filled. There is no standard data source to provide comparison prices when creating the base fee for such new tests. What private health plans pay for a new laboratory test is generally considered proprietary information and frequently is not available to the carriers because of firewalls between their private and government business. Also, some private payers may wait to see the price Medicare sets before calculating their own fee.

For these new gap-fill tests, HCFA relies on the carriers to set their own fees for the first year after it has approved coverage. HCFA specifies which new CPT codes are to be gap-filled by the carrier with the issuance of each new fee schedule, but it does not tell the carriers how to calculate the payment amount.

There is much flexibility in the way each carrier collects information and sets its fees. All 56 carriers go through the gap-fill exercise separately, in order to develop their area-specific fee for the test being added to the fee schedule. The carrier medical directors and their advisory committees may attempt to analyze the steps, methods, and materials that are used in the test in order to collect relevant cost data. Manufacturers of the new technology may be willing to provide an analysis of the costs involved with conducting the new test. Carrier medical directors are rarely pathologists and the quality of the gap-fill analyses may reflect the level of clinical laboratory expertise available within the carrier. Also, a number of carriers have consultants to help in this process, and some carriers survey laboratories for their pricing.

Charge data are not always available on new tests so carriers attempt to collect cost data in addition to prices paid by other insurers, where available. On occasion it has been necessary for HCFA to continue the carriers' fees for a second year in gap-fill status for a particularly problematic test, such as the HIV viral load, because extra time was required to collect data for setting the fee. There appears to be no attempt to collect cost data on a national basis for the new tests, or to share the data collected among several carriers or even within a single carrier that covers more than one area. Variations in the price-setting methodologies of carriers and in the fees calculated seem to be encouraged by

HCFA. While there are limited written instructions on gap-filling (and none specifically relate to laboratory tests), HCFA staff has informally stressed the need for independent cost analyses because it wants each area to develop its own fee, reflective of the local area's economy. In addition, HCFA wants a spread of fees among the 56 carriers from which it selects the median for calculating the NLA. While HCFA does not discourage the sharing of technical information about the nature of the new technology among carriers, the carriers generally appear to work independently on the gap-fill process.

There are two distinct problems with gap-filling that can sometimes lead to setting inappropriate payment levels. First, carriers set their fees based on historical experience, current cost data, and analysis, but unless they inflate the fees before the NLA is applied, it could create payments that are substantially below costs. This occurs because of the nature of the mandated formula, which sets the level of the NLA at 74 percent of the median of the carriers' gap-fill fees. The second problem is that there is no mechanism for reassessing the appropriateness of the NLA and revising a gap-fill fee once the NLA has been set. Even if the cost of the new test drops significantly after it comes into common use and may become easier to conduct, or even if the gap-fill fee is so low it could limit availability, there is no routine and practical method for changing it. Hence, neither HCFA nor the carriers regularly look back at fees set earlier to see if they are still reasonable.

As an indication of how frequently the gap-fill process is used, during 2000, carriers were required to gap-fill 13 codes and provide their fees to HCFA by May 2000 (HCFA, 1999). HCFA will then calculate the NLAs for the 2001 fee schedule. Because of numerous new CPT codes added in 1993 there were 98 gap-fills. Since then, there has been an average of 13 new gap-fills annually.

Updating Payments

Payments are rarely constant over time. Depending on the payment methodology and base, either providers or payers can raise payments. In the case of charge-based payment, providers initiate payment growth through higher charges. In other cases, when providers and payers renegotiate annual contracts, they may change the level of payment based, for example, on information about input cost increases, productivity changes, case-mix changes, quality considerations, or administrative processes. Medicare's two more mature prospective payment systems, the hospital prospective payment system (PPS) and the physician fee schedule, both rely on administratively set update amounts that are supposed to reflect similar sets of legislatively prescribed factors.[12]

---

[12]The process of developing and recommending update factors is discussed in the March annual reports of the Physician Payment Review Commission (PPRC, 1990) by the Prospective Payment Assessment Commission (1991, pp. 30–31). The process for the Medicare Fee Schedule is also described in the PPRC (1997) report to Congress.

For laboratory payments, beginning in 1984, each carrier calculated its own fee schedule using its 1983 prevailing charges at the 60 percent level plus an annual inflation factor. Originally, the inflation factor used was the urban CPI. After four years, Congress reduced the update rate—in some years to slightly less than the CPI, in other years to zero (Table 4.1). The President's original budget proposal for FY 2001 included an annual update of Medicare's laboratory fee schedule for fiscal years 2003 through 2005 of the CPI minus 1 percent. The administration estimated this would save the federal government $180 million.

As with the setting of the NLA levels, the update provides Congress with a mechanism to help control Medicare spending. If Congress thinks laboratory payments are excessive, either because new technology is perceived to have substantially lowered the cost of producing many tests or because other payers are paying less than Medicare, it can simply reduce the update. The combination of the reductions in NLAs and limited inflation updates has contributed to a recent reduction in total Medicare outpatient clinical laboratory spending in real dollars.

Adjustments

It may be appropriate to adjust payments for certain circumstances associated with measurable cost differences in the provision of services that are important to the payer. Alternatively, it may be appropriate to provide an adjustment to encourage a particular behavior that is considered beneficial in terms of explicit policy objectives. Some adjustments may occur naturally in retrospective, cost-based systems since these types of payments can reflect the costs of the specific characteristics of the service provided. Charge-based systems might also implicitly reflect variations in particular factors.

In a PPS, however, such adjustments have to be accounted for more explicitly. Potential factors for which adjustments may be appropriate include site of care, local input price variation, differences in patient health status or risk, access goals, or other payer goals. Adjustments can apply to both fee-for-service and capitated payments. Currently, the Medicare laboratory fee schedule has two adjustments built into the current system: (1) a geographic adjustment and (2) a sole community hospital adjustment.

Geographic Adjustment

There is no explicit geographic adjuster in the current laboratory payment methodology because it is inherent in the use of 56 state-based carrier fee schedules. Whatever geographic variations in charges existed in 1983 have been carried forward with various updates for inflation. The committee was unable to find evidence concerning whether charge variations from state to state were related to cost variations. Over time, the geographic disparity among the 56 fee schedules has been muted by the imposition of NLAs.

The committee examined the spread of carrier fees to determine the amount of variation from carrier to carrier. It is impossible to know whether this spread is indicative of cost differences. However, nearly 40 percent of the values in carrier fee schedules vary by more than 25 percent (either above or below) from the relevant service median value. Those that fall sufficiently below the median will be paid at rates below the NLAs, while all of those above 74 percent of the median will be paid at the NLAs, reducing the effective geographic differences in payments. Only 16 percent of service payment amounts are less than the NLAs. The amount of variation in payments is not as broad as that of the carrier fees because the NLAs cap all carrier fees that would be above them (Appendix B).

Sole Community Hospital Adjustment

Fees for laboratories based in qualified sole community hospitals currently receive a special adjustment.[13] Each year, the new fee schedules are published at the 60 percent level with separate instructions to carriers on how to calculate the fees at 62 percent for the qualified hospitals in their area. There are two additional adjustments that can be applied when payment amounts are inappropriate, but they are used only on rare occasions.

Base-Fee Adjustment

If a carrier sees a major problem with a particular fee being too low (often identified by the test's manufacturer) or, less likely, too high, it can ask the HCFA policy office for an adjustment. This happens rarely, for an obviously aberrant situation perhaps based on "data errors" or historical happenstance. Also, a representative from the laboratory or medical device industry (often with the support of members of Congress) may ask for an adjustment to the base fee of a particular test. There are only one or two such requests each year. In those cases in which HCFA decides to adjust the fee, it does so either as the whole schedule is being updated or on an interim basis by substituting the national median for the carrier's fee. Use of the national median avoids the need to recalculate the current NLA and pricing amounts for all carriers. There are no public guidelines describing this adjustment process, but program memos were issued to carriers in the mid-1990s explaining how to apply for such an adjustment. Now, HCFA solicits comments (on the fee schedule in general) each December through a program memorandum to its contractors when it posts the new fee schedule and the accompanying explanatory program memorandum on its Web

---

[13]A sole community hospital is located 25–35 miles from similar hospitals, serves at least 75 percent of the local residents needing such inpatient care, and meets the detailed criteria contained in 42 C.F.R. 412.92. A qualified hospital laboratory in a sole community hospital is one that provides some clinical diagnostic tests 24 hours a day, seven days a week, in order to serve the hospital's emergency room, which is also available around the clock.

site. Since the fee schedule takes effect on January 1 of each year, comments are reviewed and necessary changes take effect in the following year's schedule.

Inherent Reasonableness

The Secretary of DHHS has the authority to adjust payments for particular items and services paid under Part B that are considered to be "grossly excessive or grossly deficient, . . . not inherently reasonable" (COBRA). HCFA interpreted this provision as codifying both its authority and that of its carriers to establish realistic and equitable payment amounts. Complex consultative and regulatory requirements make the process cumbersome and extremely lengthy. For this reason, HCFA has attempted to adjust only one fee, not from the outpatient clinical laboratory system. Although the BBA expanded the Secretary's authority for inherent reasonableness to include outpatient clinical laboratory fees and simplified the process, it has yet to be applied. The proposed process allows consideration of issues such as whether the payment amount reflects changing technology, increased facility with that technology, or reductions in acquisition or production costs; the Medicare amount is substantially higher or lower than the payment made for the item or service by other purchasers; the marketplace is not competitive; there are grossly inappropriate geographic variations in payment amounts; and there have been increases in payment amounts that cannot be explained by inflation or technology.

Opposition from the provider community prompted a congressional request for a study by the General Accounting Office and a moratorium on inherent reasonableness adjustments until the report was released. The report supported use of the expedited system, once criteria and procedures have been clarified (GAO, 2000). It will be necessary for the Secretary to publish a final rule responding to the GAO report before the process can be implemented.

An alternative approach to adjusting specific test fees, which has been used by the administration as well as the laboratory industry, is through Congress' changing fees legislatively. Such changes to specific test fees are discussed in the preceding section on level of payment.

Cost Sharing

Payers typically include some form of cost sharing to reduce the chance that patients seek unnecessary or ineffective care.[14] There are several different mechanisms that affect how much a patient may pay for covered health services. First, some insurance policies include a deductible, so the patient is responsible for all provider charges until the deductible is met. Second, policies include copayments, also called coinsurance, which might range from a fixed, relatively

---

[14]See Phelps (1997, pp. 119–133) for an economic explanation of alternative cost-sharing approaches and their effect on service use.

small dollar amount within a managed care plan to a percentage of the provider's charges in a fee-for-service plan. Third, providers may ask patients to pay any charges in excess of those covered by the payer. This balance may be quite large if the payer approves only a small percentage of the provider's charges and there are no limits on how much the provider may charge the patient.

Copayments and deductibles are commonly used in the Medicare program. For Medicare physician services, for example, beneficiaries pay 20 percent of the Medicare Fee Schedule amount and the program pays the other 80 percent. The laboratory payment system is unusual because it includes no beneficiary cost sharing.

EFFECT OF LABORATORY SPENDING ON PHYSICIAN PAYMENT

Aggregate Medicare spending for laboratory services influences Medicare physician fees. The volume of laboratory services is included in the measure of physician service volume that is incorporated into the sustainable growth rate (SGR) used to calculate the annual update factor for the Medicare Fee Schedule for physicians' services (Balanced Budget Act of 1997, Public Law 105-33).

Unexpected growth in the volume of laboratory services may affect Medicare's spending for laboratory services directly, but its effect on total Medicare spending is muted because spending on physicians' services can be controlled. If, for example, laboratory service volumes grew faster than expected, physician payment rates would be updated by less than would have occurred with lower laboratory volumes. As a result, with spending for laboratory services growing faster than expected (in this hypothetical example), physician spending would be slowed, insulating total Medicare spending from the growth in laboratory expenditures. The inclusion of laboratory services in the calculation of physician payment updates recognizes the role of physicians in determining the volume of laboratory services used by beneficiaries. The SGR applies only to physician payments and does not affect the outpatient clinical laboratory payment methodology, the calculation of laboratory payment rates, or Medicare spending on laboratory services in any way.

CONCLUSION

This chapter has examined the elements of the Medicare clinical laboratory payment system in some detail. Although these elements have been described individually, they do not operate in isolation: the functioning of one element affects others. Also, the laboratory payment system, as a whole, does not operate in isolation. Other regulatory and market mechanisms affect the operation of the payment methodology. Considering the various payment elements of the current system discussed in this chapter and their interrelationships with the external forces discussed in Chapters 2 and 3 is important for assessing the current system and considering alternatives.

REFERENCES

Committee on Ways and Means, U.S. House of Representatives. 1998. *1998 Green Book: Overview of Entitlement Programs*. Washington, DC: U.S. Government Printing Office.

Government Accounting Office (GAO). 2000. *Medicare Payments: Use of Revised "Inherent Reasonableness" Process Generally Appropriate*. HEHS-00-79. Washington, DC: GAO.

HCFA. 1999. Program Memorandum: Transmittal No. AB-99-84; Subject: Implementation of Calendar Year (CY) 2000 Clinical Diagnostic Laboratory Fee Schedule and Laboratory and Ambulance Costs Subject to Reasonable Charge Payment Methodology in 2000. Web page, accessed September 5, 2000. Available at http://www.hcfa.gov/pubforms/transmit/AB998460.htm.

HCFA. 2000a. Proposed Rule: Medicare Program; Negotiated Rulemaking: Coverage and Administrative Policies for Clinical Diagnostic Laboratory Services. *Federal Register* 65, No. 48:13082–13167.

HCFA. 2000b. FY 2000 Clinical Diagnostic Laboratory Fee Schedule. Web page, accessed January 3, 2000. Available at http://www.hcfa.gov/stats/cpt/clfdown.htm.

Lewin Group, Inc. 2000. *Outlook for medical technology innovation: Will patients get the care they need? Report 2: The Medicare payment process and patient access to technology*, Washington, DC: The Health Industry Manufacturers Association.

Logue, J. 1996. Federal reimbursement to laboratories. *Clin Chem* 42, No. 5:817–821.

Medicare Payment Advisory Commission (MedPAC). 1998. *Report to the Congress: Medicare Payment Policy 1998*. Washington, DC: MedPAC.

Medicare Program; Procedures for Making National Coverage Decisions. 1999. *Federal Register* 64, No. 80:22619–22625.

Medicare Program; Criteria for Making Coverage Decisions. 2000. *Federal Register* 65, No. 95:31124–31129.

Merrell, K. 2000. Paying for Clinical Laboratory Services under Medicare: Framework for Describing and Assessing Policy Options (unpublished). Chicago, IL.

Phelps, C. E. 1997. *Health Economics, Second Edition*. Reading, MA: Addision-Wesley.

Physician Payment Review Commission (PPRC). 1990. *Annual Report to Congress 1990*. Washington, D.C.: PPRC.

PPRC. 1992. *Annual Report to Congress 1992*. Washington, D.C.: PPRC.

PPRC. 1993. *Annual Report to Congress 1993*. Washington, D.C.: PPRC.

PPRC. 1997. *Basics,* No. 6, September. Washington, D.C.: PPRC.

Prospective Payment Assessment Commission. 1991. *Report and Recommendations to the Congress*. Washington, D.C.: Prospective Payment Assessment Commission.

Silva, C. May 23, 2000. FDA: Moving forward with CLIA 88. Hunt Valley, MD: *CLMA Annual Laboratory Seminar 2000*.

5
The Current System: How Well Does It Work?

The committee concluded that the current Medicare payment methodology is functioning well enough to achieve the crucial goal of unhindered beneficiary access to outpatient clinical laboratory services. It also concluded that some of the administrative complexities of the payment methodology are financially wasteful and harmful to laboratory services providers. The committee's examination revealed significant problems and considerable room for improving the system.

The committee gathered information to determine how well the current system meets the goals identified in Chapter 1. Unfortunately, the information is quite limited. Much of it came from stakeholders and other parties involved with laboratory services.

BENEFICIARY ACCESS

The committee found no evidence that beneficiaries have difficulty obtaining outpatient clinical laboratory services.

There appear to be adequate numbers of laboratories and specimen collection stations so that beneficiaries are receiving needed services. The committee looked for evidence of even limited access problems, even if the causes could not be clearly attributed to the payment method.

General Access. The current geographic locations, number of sites, and capacity of the laboratories provide access for beneficiaries.

The committee found no evidence that beneficiaries or physicians are encountering difficulties in obtaining needed laboratory tests. The Health Care Financing Administration (HCFA) has not received any complaints about access problems. Laboratory services are not a significant concern of consumer groups that speak for Medicare beneficiaries. There is no evidence of even limited problems, for example, in rural areas.

The number of laboratories has increased nationally since the fee schedule was established in 1984. A study by the Office of the Inspector General (OIG) assessed the impact of the Clinical Laboratory Improvement Amendments of 1988 (CLIA) on the number of laboratories, and their distribution, with particular attention to rural areas. In 1995, CLIA had issued 151,658 certificates for laboratories, including multiple certificates for the same site—for example, two or more separate laboratories located at the same hospital center. In its analysis, which counted only one of the multiple laboratories located at the same site, the OIG found an average of 51 clinical laboratories for every 100,000 persons and nearly one site for every four physicians. Of the more than 3,000 counties in the country, only 66 had no laboratory site (38 of these had no physician medical practice site). Rural counties had nearly the same number of laboratories per capita as non-rural counties (OIG, 1995).

Between 1985 and 1995, the number of Medicare beneficiaries increased by less than 3 percent a year. The number of laboratory tests performed on beneficiaries grew an average of 17 percent annually (OIG, 1995). The OIG found no evidence of an insufficient supply of laboratories or access problems. Between 1995 and March 2000, the number of CLIA-certified laboratories nationally grew from 151,658 (including multisite laboratories if registered or certified separately) to 170,000 (Dyckman and Cassidy, 2000).

Although approximately 5,000 short-stay hospitals participate in Medicare (HCFA, 1998), there are currently 8,560 hospital-based laboratories, almost 5,000 independent laboratory sites, and 105,000 physician office laboratories (POLs) certified by CLIA (Table 2.1). Virtually all participate in Medicare. The committee found no evidence that POLs are denying access to Medicare beneficiaries, that beneficiaries are having difficulty finding a POL, or that physicians have reduced access since 1995.

For beneficiaries who have difficulty reaching one of the 170,000 certified laboratories, independent laboratories run specimen collection stations.[1] At such stations, there are staff who draw and collect specimens and transport them to the laboratory that performs the tests. Often the test is run overnight, and the physician has the results in the morning. Similarly, most physicians, even if they do not have a laboratory in their office, generally are willing to have their staff collect specimens for the convenience of their patients. A laboratory service picks up the specimens from the physician's office on a daily basis. Collection

---

[1]Because these stations are not certified under CLIA, there are no federal statistics available on their numbers.

stations and physicians' offices significantly expand the options available to beneficiaries seeking access to laboratory services.

Financial Access. The Medicare program imposes no financial barriers to outpatient clinical laboratory services for beneficiaries.

Unlike other Part B services and supplies, there are no financial barriers for the beneficiary. Copayments and deductibles for laboratory services were eliminated in 1984. The President's budget for FY 2001 proposed to reimpose the Part B 20 percent copayment for laboratory tests. The explanation given for including this proposal in the administration's budget was to rationalize ". . . current cost sharing requirements. . . ," to help finance benefit improvements, and ". . . to prevent over-utilization and reduce fraud. . . " (Executive Office of the President, 2000).

The administration's proposed budget for FY 2001 projects $2.4 billion in Medicare savings (2001–2005) from the laboratory copayment proposal. The $2.4 billion in savings is expected to accrue mainly from Medicare paying laboratories at 80 percent of the carrier's fee or the National Limitation Amount (NLA), whichever is lower. Medicare will also generate savings indirectly, from reduced payments for managed care beneficiaries because of lower fee-for-service spending.[2] HCFA actuaries concluded that only a small, unspecified fraction of the savings would come from reduced utilization. Although the $2.4 billion in savings may materialize, it does not translate into the same amount of savings for the health system, because laboratories would bear an extra expense to bill beneficiaries for copayments and would likely accumulate bad debt.

The fees for many laboratory tests are relatively low. The average fee for the top 100 tests by dollar volume was about $11.00 in 1998. A 20 percent copayment averages less than $2.30. A typical medical visit that results in lab tests includes only a modest number of tests. In some laboratories the average is 2.5 tests per claim. The cost to the laboratory is relatively high for billing the copayment and often would exceed the amount of money the laboratory would receive, even if all copayments were collected, since generating and sending a business letter is estimated to cost more than $5.

Access to STAT Tests. The committee found no evidence that Medicare beneficiaries are being denied STAT (literally, at once) tests when medically indicated.

There is obvious value to having access to test results quickly or almost instantly. Fast turnaround can mean starting the correct treatment sooner, convenience for the beneficiary, possibly a better treatment outcome, and potential cost savings. Under emergency conditions, STAT tests are essential and can mean

[2] The Medicare formula for capitation payments to managed care organizations is tied, in part, to per capita spending for fee-for-service beneficiaries (MedPac, 1999).

the difference between life and death. Hospitals, particularly those with emergency rooms, must maintain the capacity to produce STAT results for patients with emergency conditions. In addition, as discussed in Chapter 3, many facilities are acquiring equipment to provide tests at the point of care. The extra 2 percent payment for qualified sole community provider hospitals offers some compensation for the extra standby capacity.

Testimony to the committee indicated that laboratories could incur additional costs when they do a STAT test because the laboratory interrupts the routine of its staff and equipment. Sometimes expensive test kits designed for multiple specimens are wasted when only one segment is used for a STAT test. Hospital and emergency facility laboratories must staff to be able to perform STAT tests at all hours. The committee is not aware of any studies that systematically identify which tests might prove cost-effective when done on an expedited basis and under what circumstances.

The committee found no evidence of restricted access to STAT tests for beneficiaries, even though Medicare laboratory payments do not distinguish between tests conducted STAT and those done with a 24-hour turnaround time or longer. Laboratories are all paid the same amount for the same test, regardless of turnaround time, by many private as well as public insurers. The committee notes, however, that some private payers do pay additional sums for tests (and other medical services) done on an emergency basis. The Current Procedural Terminology (CPT) Editorial Panel has not supported the use of code modifiers to report the emergency nature of medical services generally. For laboratory tests, specifically, the American Medical Association (AMA) does not consider a special code for STAT services appropriate, because STAT tests are considered a normal part of medical practice as are other emergency medical services.

FLEXIBILITY

The committee concluded that existing mechanisms are inadequate for keeping payments up to date. The inflation factor and the NLA level raise or lower fees across the board for all tests but do not provide adjustments to accommodate changes needed in payment levels for specific tests. The process for integrating new technologies into the payment system, including determinations of coverage, assignment of billing codes, and development of appropriate prices, is slow, administratively inefficient, and closed to stakeholder participation. These problems are likely to become increasingly important with the anticipated changes in laboratory technology and medical practice.

The growing number of laboratories indicates that Medicare beneficiaries are receiving the care they need and suggests that the payment system has adapted sufficiently to continue functioning in changing times.

Formal Mechanisms. As discussed in Chapter 4, some mechanisms permit adaptation to changes in the Medicare budget, financial environment, and technology. The size of the inflation factor for updating the carriers' fee schedules is determined by the Congress during the budget reconciliation process. It can be set to reflect changes in the general economy or in general input costs for producing laboratory services. Congress can also use this mechanism to adjust federal budget exigencies, setting the update rate above or below the level of inflation.

Congressional authority to set the level of the NLAs (the percentage of the median of the carriers' fees to be used as a cap) constitutes another payment adjustment mechanism. It can be used to raise or lower the national caps on all fees across the board. This provided a means to address concerns that Medicare payments for laboratory tests were generally much higher than laboratory charges to physicians for the same tests.

There are several other problems, however, that the system has not addressed. Since laboratory charges in 1983 were not linked to costs, some Medicare test fees, which were based on those charges, are inappropriately high or low. Additionally, both changes in technology that have made some testing techniques more efficient, and advances that have improved quality but cost more, have further skewed relationships between costs and payments. Adjustment of the inflation factor and the NLA level cannot remedy the problems of fees for individual tests. The "inherent reasonableness" mechanism was designed to modify fees that are grossly out of line. Unfortunately, this mechanism has been so impracticable that it has hardly been used at the national level. A recent General Accounting Office (GAO) report concerning durable medical equipment (DME) and supplies supports HCFA's use of an expedited inherent reasonableness process, which could be used for laboratory fees as well (GAO, 2000). Once the final regulation for an expedited process is promulgated, it could provide a more practical approach for adjusting individual test fees.

Sometimes the Congress has been asked to change particular fees that the laboratory industry or HCFA has considered too low or too high. For example, the 106th Congress raised the fee for certain Pap smears, and the administration asked Congress in its 2001 budget to reduce the fees for four other high-volume tests. These political interventions are not an efficient way to deal with individual test fees. HCFA needs mechanisms that operate on a regular review cycle, allow for off-cycle consideration of problems, and include input from various stakeholders and experts to provide validity and flexibility to the process.

Coverage Changes. Over time, changes in medical practice affect the payment system. The recent negotiated rulemaking on coverage policies for laboratory tests is an attempt to move the payment system toward more evidenced-based coverage policies. It established a five-year cycle for review of national policies. If the committee's recommendation on the use of the International Classification of Diseases, Ninth Revision (ICD-9) codes for prepayment review is implemented, it would be necessary to reconsider the use of such coverage policies.

New Technology. The incorporation of new technology into the Medicare outpatient laboratory payment system is an important challenge for three reasons: (1) the current fee schedule is based on laboratory charges in 1983; (2) many new tests, methods, and equipment developed since 1983 are not in the Medicare base year charge data; and (3) the rate of development of new testing technologies is growing.

The process for incorporating innovation, including Food and Drug Administration (FDA) approval of a new technology, assignment of a code, determination of coverage by Medicare, and development of fees through cross-walk and gap-fill procedures, is considered problematic by stakeholders. Even the Congress criticized HCFA for not incorporating particular new technologies (for screening Pap smears) quickly enough (Congressional Record, H12512, Public Law 106-113, section 224). The committee could find no studies on Medicare's impact on technological innovation or the availability of new technologies to beneficiaries, compared to other health plans. The committee did learn that some private payers wait until Medicare makes coverage decisions and sets fees for new technology before making their own decisions (Appendix C). It is clear, however, that HCFA's method for setting fees for new tests is flawed. Some specific concerns about the current methods for incorporating new technologies into the payment system include the following:

- The process for deciding which tests and technologies are cross-walked or gap-filled is not publicly explained, based on published criteria, or inclusive of stakeholders.
- There is a duplicative, decentralized process for collecting data for gap filling that does not offer written instructions specifically relating to laboratory services for the carriers and has little public involvement.
- The legislatively mandated formula for calculating gap-fill test fees is likely to result in prices that are too low relative to costs because HCFA is required to base the NLA on 74 percent of the median of the 56 carriers' fees. If the 56 carriers' fees accurately reflect costs, then the NLA is likely to be unreasonably low.

TRANSPARENCY

The committee concluded that the current payment system lacks "openness" and adequate procedures for stakeholder involvement. Clear and consistent information on how the system works and opportunities for the public and stakeholders to have input into decision processes are limited.

The committee heard frequent complaints from the industry that it was unclear how carriers determined gap-fill fees, set claims-processing review procedures, and established local medical review policies (LMRPs). In addition, the industry questioned how HCFA decided which new tests should be cross-walked or gap-filled and how the cross-walk code was selected. Some expressed the view that these processes could benefit from public input. Greater opportunity for stakeholder input could also bring additional useful information into the process.

Publicly available clarifications of these procedures could improve provider compliance and reduce mistakes in claims submissions. Public input to policies and procedures is limited, particularly compared to the openness of the recent negotiated rulemaking exercise on national coverage policies.

A number of recent improvements may increase transparency. All LMRPs for Medicare carriers are now available through the Web. This service would be more helpful to interested providers if the Web site were easier to use and if it were kept current. The negotiated rulemaking on coverage addressed several provider concerns—for example, the use of frequency criteria to deny claims for selected tests on grounds of medical necessity. Once the rule takes effect, contractors will be required to publish frequency limits for particular tests before they apply the limits in processing claims.

VALUE

The committee found it had little data with which to judge whether Medicare spending in aggregate is too high or too low, whether Medicare is paying reasonable amounts for individual tests and services, or whether physicians are ordering tests appropriately. The committee concluded that Medicare purchases tests that meet Medicare standards for its beneficiaries with minimal or no beneficiary access problems. Medicare payments appear to be within the range of private payments.

Paying the Right Amount. At the individual test level, it is unclear whether Medicare payments represent good value. The current payment system is based on historical charges, which may or may not reflect costs. An extensive search found no comprehensive, representative, reliable data on current or historical costs for the production of laboratory tests. The committee also has no basis for judging whether the current relationship between the fees for individual tests and their costs of production creates financial disincentives for physicians to order medically appropriate tests. The payment survey conducted for this study showed that Medicare fees for 22 selected, high-volume services fell within the range of payments used by several Blue Cross plans. Although the data are not conclusive, they do indicate comparability among fee schedules (Appendix C).

The committee is unable to assess if the current NLA could be lowered further without jeopardizing beneficiary access. Similarly, there is no empirical basis to support claims by the laboratory industry that the NLA needs to be raised. The number of laboratories is growing, which implies that excessively low Medicare payments are not driving laboratories from the market.

When examining new laboratory technologies, there is no mechanism within the current payment system and related regulatory processes that encourages consideration of the costs and benefits of covering new tests. Hence, new tests are added to the laboratory fee schedules without consideration of their cost-effectiveness relative to existing tests. In certain narrowly defined cases, this may change, if new coverage criteria now under consideration are implemented. Once a test is approved for coverage, a fee is set, but the current payment method does not necessarily result in a price that accurately reflects the costs of performing the test initially or over time.

Fraud and Abuse. Fraud and abuse lower the value of aggregate Medicare spending for laboratory services. The payment system, along with other aspects of the program, can affect the extent of fraud and abuse. The OIG considers clinical laboratory services particularly vulnerable to fraud, waste, and abuse. One indicator of value is the extent of such problems in the payment system. Some of the OIG's largest civil settlements (hundreds of millions of dollars) are related to Medicare payments to clinical laboratory companies. According to the OIG, many fraudulent practices in the laboratory industry have been addressed in the past few years. The cases of fraud and abuse were not prevented, detected, or corrected through mechanisms within the Medicare payment system. Rather, they were identified by whistle-blowers and audits and dealt with through corporate integrity agreements, voluntary compliance plans, and legal proceedings. The OIG asserted that the inadequate controls used by contractors to detect and prevent inappropriate payments and the lack of any financial involvement and oversight by beneficiaries contributed to circumstances that have encouraged fraud and abuse.

ADMINISTRATIVE SIMPLICITY AND EFFICIENCY

> *The committee concluded that administration of the Medicare outpatient laboratory payment system, with its 56 separate fee schedules and 56 separate processes for coverage determination, is unnecessarily complex and inefficient, particularly in the way the system incorporates new technologies and determines whether or not a laboratory's claim should be paid.*

Number of Carrier Jurisdictions. Since most of the individual test fees on the 56 separate fee schedules are close to the NLA, the administrative value of the original system is now greatly diminished. In fact, the committee believes it creates more confusion and administrative work than it is worth. Similarly, the existence of 56 sets of LMRPs creates confusion and administrative burdens for physicians, laboratories, and conceivably even beneficiaries because of overlap in the tests to which these policies apply, some overlap in definitions of medically necessary codes, and sometimes widely divergent lists of acceptable diagnosis codes. As with the 56 fee schedules, there is little justification for creating different LMRPs for each of the 56 jurisdictions.

New Technology. The gap-fill process for calculating new test fees suffers from inadequate administrative guidance and inefficiencies. The lack of guidance on how to analyze new technologies—what data to use, acceptable methodologies for estimating costs, and approaches to break down the scientific testing methods—ensures inconsistent analyses of varying quality and differing prices that are not necessarily related to actual costs. With additional guidance from HCFA, each carrier could perhaps conduct these gap-fill analyses more efficiently, but the greater waste is having the 56 carriers each doing separate analyses. Given the number of gap-fills each year, an average of 13 per year from 1994 to 2000, considerable staff effort and expertise is required. There is little reason to expect drastically different costs beyond differences attributable to geographic price variations and rates of diffusion.[3]

Claims Denials. The fact that 15 percent of the claims for the 100 highest-volume Medicare outpatient laboratory codes are denied by carriers is an indication of significant waste (Appendix E).[4] There are various reasons for denying claims, discussed in Chapter 4, in addition to the lack of medical necessity. If some claims are paid after two or more submissions and others are never paid, there is substantial wasted effort on the part of the laboratory, physician, and contractor, compared with filing and processing the claim correctly the first time or knowing not to submit it at all. The requirements for documentation of medical necessity and processing of claims denials affect not only operational efficiency, but also the cost of providing laboratory services and aggregate Medicare payments to laboratories.

The committee heard testimony that claims denials are a major frustration for the laboratory industry in dealing with Medicare. The committee could not locate any national data to show whether or not dealing with Medicare is more burdensome than dealing with other payers.

The financial burden of all denials of payments, including those based on medical necessity grounds, falls upon the laboratory, not the physician who ordered the test.[5] Likewise, it appears unfair to make the laboratory absorb the costs of performing a screening test (e.g., a Pap smear) in a circumstance in which adequate ICD-9 documentation is present, but unbeknownst to the laboratory and perhaps to the physician, the time since the last test was conducted is insufficient to meet coverage criteria. An Advanced Beneficiary Notice (ABN) is supposed to relieve the laboratory of this burden (making the patient responsible for payment when Medicare denies the claim); however, if the physician did not take the time to obtain a signed ABN, the laboratory is still responsible for

---

[3]New tests will usually be more expensive to perform when they are first marketed because they may diffuse slowly and be conducted in smaller volume.

[4]Data were not available on the denial rates of the fiscal intermediaries.

[5]Laboratories are not precluded from billing physicians for denied claims, but most are reluctant to do so because they see the physicians as customers, may assume it would not be cost-effective, or are unsure whether they could sustain a legal challenge.

the bill. Currently, the ABN process is complex and time-consuming, often requiring several minutes for a conscientious physician to help the patient understand the situation. The committee realizes that changes in the ABN form and process are under consideration and urges that any changes made be consistent with the goals of administrative simplicity and efficiency.

The committee is concerned about the national, aggregate carrier denial rate of approximately 15 percent for all tests; however, it is particularly concerned with the variation in denial rates among carriers and across specific tests that, in some cases, amounts to more than 50 percent. Variation in denial rates is attributable, in part, to geographic variations in medical practice, patient needs, fraud and abuse, coverage policies, and claims processing systems among contractors. The committee was able to obtain data from HCFA specifying the grounds for claims denials only from POL claims, which showed that only 2.5 percent of POL claims were denied because they were found to be medically unnecessary. The committee heard testimony that claims-processing procedures can vary among carriers, in part because of unclear or missing instructions from HCFA and differing interpretations of instructions. If these explanations are significant causes of variations in denial rates within and among carriers, they suggest inefficient and ineffective administration.

Medical Necessity. The committee finds that the use of ICD-9 codes as a basis for determining medical necessity is not only administratively cumbersome, but also ineffective. Under current law, the Medicare program is obligated to pay for items and services that are reasonable and necessary for the diagnosis or treatment of illness or injury unless Congress explicitly excluded them from coverage. Currently, HCFA's main method for determining the medical necessity of reasonable, covered outpatient clinical laboratory services is to have its contractors perform computerized, pre-payment screening of the laboratory service claim form for particular ICD-9 diagnosis and symptom codes that are considered by the contractor to provide an indication of the medical necessity of particular lab tests. Although such use is a well intended attempt to prevent waste and fraud and promote higher quality care, the committee finds that it has undesirable and unintended consequences.

In practice, if a claim for a laboratory service lacks an ICD-9 code that is among those that the local contractor considers to be evidence of the medical necessity for a particular test, the contractor's computer system will deny payment for the test. While the diagnosis code is required generally on all Medicare claims, it appears to be used for pre-payment screening much more commonly for laboratory services than for physician services. HCFA can not identify what percent of laboratory claims are denied by pre-payment screening on medical necessity grounds, but testimony from the industry identified it as substantial and a major cost and frustration for the laboratories.

The variations from carrier to carrier in what constitutes an acceptable ICD-9 code for a particular laboratory test add to the complexity of billing by providers that receive samples from more than one carrier area. To help providers, some commercial software companies have designed billing software that flags laboratory test codes that require specific diagnosis codes for payment. Some laboratories highlight tests with an LMRP and provide the most common, acceptable diagnoses right on their claim form to help the physician. There is a fine line between such educational or administrative assistance and gaming the system.

Because the contractors process claims for billions of laboratory tests, it seems administratively efficient to employ computerized screens for medical necessity. When only the ICD-9 code is used to determine the medical necessity of a laboratory test, however, an erroneous conclusion often may be drawn. Not only might it be wrong when it is used to conclude that a particular test is not medically necessary for a given patient (a false negative determination), but it also might be wrong when it is used to conclude that a test is medically necessary for a patient (a false positive determination). In technical terms the current approach is neither sensitive nor specific and may often be inaccurate.

During the development of local and national medical review policies, committees attempt to identify all symptoms and diagnoses that might justify the ordering of a particular laboratory test. Although these symptoms and diagnoses may justify use of a particular test in some instances, it is not necessarily the case that they would justify the ordering of a particular test in all patients who have one of those symptoms or diagnoses. For example, the medical review policy for the measurement of the blood glucose level proposed in the Neg Reg process includes many symptoms and diagnoses that may be associated with diabetes, such as senile cataract and chronic bronchitis. In fact, it is much more likely that a person who has one of these associated diseases does not have diabetes than it is for such a person to have diabetes. Thus, in most instances, the fact that a patient has one of these associated diseases is not a good indication that the determination of a blood glucose level is medically appropriate. It is impossible to use an ICD-9 code approach to establish medical necessity with any degree of confidence in its accuracy.

Although contractors do permit denied claims to be resubmitted with a different diagnosis code or additional information to justify the medical necessity of the test for a particular patient, in reality resubmission often is not administratively feasible and, hence, frequently is not attempted. Although pre-payment screening may be administratively convenient for the contractor, it is administratively burdensome for the laboratory, which must seek the information from the physician. Because the administrative costs of obtaining such information from the ordering physician may be high compared to the revenue that would be received for performing the test, many denied claims are not pursued. In contrast, false positive pre-screening determinations (i.e. determinations that a test is medically necessary, based on an ICD-9 code, when it is not) are never identified through the screening process. In effect, the ICD-9 becomes the sole determinant of medical necessity in most cases.

Information Systems. Laboratories are particularly frustrated when claims are denied on medical necessity grounds, even though the appropriate diagnosis code for the test is included on the claim form and there is no dispute about the coverage policy itself. Apparently, some carriers' computer systems are unable to read all the diagnoses codes and match them against all of the test codes. Laboratories must resubmit the claim with a different diagnosis code at the top of the list to get a computer match with the test code. Claims with several tests and diagnoses may require multiple submissions before they are paid. This may represent a computer systems issue that could be addressed when the specifications for the regional laboratory claims processors are designed.

Local Medical Review Policies. Although not all carriers need LMRPs for the same tests, the fact that carriers often have different LMRPs covering the same tests is an indication of inefficient management.[6] Carriers decide to create an LMRP for various reasons. For example, one carrier may need a policy for a new test that is not marketed nationally, or different medical practices may lead to overuse of a particular test only in certain parts of the country. However, if the review policy is based on medical evidence, there is no justification for developing policy separately in multiple carriers instead of developing one policy at the national level and applying it in areas where needed. Also, in most cases there is no rationale for having many different ICD-9 codes approved for a test in one area but not another. The 23 national medical review policies developed under the negotiated rulemaking may eliminate many inconsistent LMRPs. Also, consolidation of the outpatient laboratory claims-processing functions into four or five regional carriers may reduce the numbers of duplicative coverage policies developed for each test and, possibly, inconsistencies among carriers, depending on how that administrative function is designed. For laboratories serving patients from multiple carrier jurisdictions, this consolidation is expected to result in a major administrative simplification.

Administrative Efficiencies. Certain aspects of the claims payment process are administered more efficiently than the concerns discussed above. HCFA reports that contractors find laboratory claims relatively easy and inexpensive to process compared to other claims. Some provider representatives point to the electronic submission of claims and payments as an advantage of the current system and certainly an improvement over the traditional paper processes.

OTHER ISSUES OF CONCERN

The committee identified several important issues that are related to, but extend beyond, the Medicare laboratory payment methodology. A responsible analysis of these issues would take the committee beyond the scope of this study

---

[6]This may also reflect the notion that local autonomy is necessary to deal with local conditions.

and beyond its charge. The committee considers these issues briefly with the expectation that others will pursue them in greater depth.

Improving the Quality and Appropriate Use of Laboratory Services

To date, most quality control and quality improvement efforts in outpatient clinical laboratory testing have focused on the laboratory itself and the accuracy of its test results. There is evidence of excessive and inappropriate use of clinical laboratory tests in the hospital inpatient setting, but there are no comparable studies of the use of laboratory tests in outpatient clinics and physicians' offices (Axt-Adam et al., 1993; Hindmarsh and Lyon, 1996; van Walraven and Naylor, 1998). The extent of inappropriate outpatient testing is unknown. While laboratories may recognize orders that might be inappropriate and may offer expert advice or educational materials to the physician, the committee found little concerted effort to improve the appropriateness of test ordering in the context of patient care.

Because laboratory payments do not represent a very large portion of the budget for Medicare, managed-care plans, third-party payers, or hospitals, these organizations have less incentive to focus on changing utilization patterns for laboratory tests than they do for other types of care. Other options to improve the quality of clinical testing require consideration:

- The Agency for Healthcare Research and Quality should support more research on the proper treatment of selected diseases and medical problems that includes attention to the use of outpatient clinical laboratory tests in the full context of medical care.
- Education for physicians by experts in the effective use of laboratory tests should target medical conditions likely to yield large returns and for which practice guidelines and scientific evidence exist. Both the public and the private sectors should encourage clinicians and laboratorians to work together to develop (1) educational materials incorporating cost-effective algorithms to improve utilization of tests, (2) assessments of tests required for specific diagnoses, and (3) care plans that include tests for the diagnosis and monitoring of the selected conditions. It is important to use educational methods that are acceptable to the audience and effective in changing practice patterns and health outcomes.
- Laboratorians and physicians should work together to conduct a systematic review of the full laboratory fee schedule to identify obsolete tests that no longer offer value and need never be used for any case. This would provide another opportunity for the various laboratory-related associations and physicians' organizations to work together to update clinical practice. New tests and testing methods are supplanting old tests and raising the quality of care, but it is difficult for physicians to keep up with all the changes. As long as obsolete tests are coded and remain on the fee schedule, some physicians will order them and some laboratories will provide them. The list of obsolete codes could be presented to the

AMA's CPT Editorial Panel for elimination from the CPT code listing. In addition, these same tests could be submitted to the local Carrier Advisory Committee for consideration of eliminating coverage for them. Once the codes are deleted and the information is clearly communicated to all stakeholders, physicians' ordering habits and laboratories' test menus would likely conform since there would no longer be a code and fee available for billing purposes.

The above measures will improve the treatment and diagnosis of all patients, not only Medicare beneficiaries, and may also save Medicare and other payers money. These efforts should be considered, regardless of the type of payment methodology Medicare uses.

Coding Process for Outpatient Laboratory Tests

The clinical laboratory industry and manufacturers of laboratory tests and equipment testified that the current process for obtaining a CPT code is cumbersome and slow. The committee recognizes that obtaining a CPT code is only one piece of the complex and lengthy process required to identify and incorporate new technology into the Medicare program, but it is worthy of examination nonetheless.

The AMA noted that the CPT code process operated on a 12-month publication cycle, but the full review and decision process to obtain a new code could take longer, depending on the timing of the submission of a coding suggestion. There should be ways to expedite this process for new technologies. Likewise, there are ways to shorten the process for incorporating new technologies into the laboratory payment system, even without coding changes, that should be undertaken in any case.[7] The committee also discussed whether CPT codes or some other coding system, such as the International Classification of Diseases, Tenth Revision (ICD-10) or CLIA systems, might be more appropriate for identifying laboratory services.

- The ICD-10 coding system is reported to be more extensive than the current ICD-9 for diagnoses and symptoms and, in the United States, will also have codes for procedures appended. Developmental work is not complete, and ICD-10 was not ready for consideration by the committee. However, HCFA should consider whether ICD-10 could be useful for identifying outpatient clinical laboratory tests as it is currently envisioned or with minor adjustments during its development. An obvious concern is how new tests and technologies would be assigned a code within the system and how long it would take.
- The CLIA coding system identifies each test, testing equipment, or methodology and categorizes it according to complexity. Since CLIA codes are assigned relatively promptly following FDA test approval, this has some advantages. Its value for claims-processing purposes has yet to be explored.

---

[7]See committee recommendations in Chapter 7.

Clearly, these coding systems were designed to serve many clinical and payment purposes beyond the needs of Medicare's clinical laboratory payment methodology. Thus, changes in the systems and processes for coding clinical laboratory services may have serious repercussions for other providers and payers as well as for clinical practice. Similarly, coding system changes undertaken for other purposes may have a significant impact on laboratory payment methodology. The committee recognizes the complexity of these coding issues and supports a thorough examination of the issues before major changes are attempted.

Fraud, Waste, and Abuse

Most providers are honest and concerned principally with the well-being of their patients. The committee realizes, however, that opportunities for fraud, waste, and abuse exist under any payment system. Some in the laboratory and physician communities may take advantage of these opportunities. Some providers quickly learn to "game the system" legally, while others step over the line with more fraudulent practices; therefore, it is important to have in place both procedures for monitoring the payment system to detect unintended consequences and strong mechanisms for detecting and preventing fraud and abuse.

- One approach to fraud detection should result from the consolidation of carriers and the creation of a Central Statistical Carrier that can provide analyses of broad trend data. The OIG expects this centralized approach to be more useful than the current system for detecting national patterns of fraud.
- Another method for detecting waste, fraud and abuse is more extensive use of focused medical reviews (FMRs) designed to identify patterns of inappropriate or unnecessary testing. The FMRs could target particular laboratories and physicians, selected geographic areas, or specific tests that are expected to yield a high return. The use of FMRs by carriers, quality improvement strategies by peer review organizations (PROs), LMRPs, and national coverage policies for prepayment and postpayment screening of claims should be compared to determine the most cost-effective methods.
- Another approach to consider is designing mechanisms to strengthen the ability of laboratories to receive compensation from the ordering physician for the costs of tests determined to be medically unnecessary or insufficiently documented.

CONCLUSION

The committee concludes that the current Medicare payment system provides adequate access for beneficiaries to outpatient clinical laboratory services, but has many problems that are likely to become more serious in the future. The system needs an appropriate, flexible mechanism for making changes in individual fees that are out of line. The system needs a more open process for developing policy and making decisions about fees and clearer communications for presenting them. Changes are also needed in administrative procedures, particularly for the incorporation of new tests, to streamline procedures and make them more efficient. The committee was concerned with the lack of data on which to base a judgment of whether HCFA's fees for individual services were set at an appropriate level and the lack of data on the frequency of inappropriate use.

The committee believes that the shortcomings discussed in this chapter can and should be addressed. Time tends to exacerbate such problems because laboratory practice and the larger health care system continue to change, thus putting further stress on an already cumbersome and inefficient system. By taking action promptly, HCFA and the Congress can revise the payment system to better accommodate the technological advances expected in the decades ahead. In the next chapter the committee discusses alternatives for change. In Chapter 7 the committee presents its recommendations for changes in payment methodology.

REFERENCES

Axt-Adam, P., J. C. van der Wouden, and E. van der Does. 1993. Influencing behavior of physicians ordering laboratory tests: A literature study. *Med Care* 31, No. 9:784–794.

Dyckman, Z., and B. B. Cassidy. 2000. Recent developments and trends in the clinical laboratory industry (unpublished). Columbia, MD: CHPS Consulting.

Executive Office of the President of the United States. 2000. *Proposed Budget of the United States Government, Fiscal Year 2001.* Washington, DC: U.S. Government Printing Office.

General Accounting Office (GAO). 2000. *Medicare Payments: Use of Revised "Inherent Reasonableness" Process Generally Appropriate.* HEHS-00-79. Washington, DC: GAO.

Health Care Financing Administration (HCFA). 1998. *1998 Data Compendium*, 030407. Baltimore, MD.: U.S. Government Printing Office.

Hindmarsh, J. T., and A. W. Lyon. 1996. Strategies to promote rational clinical chemistry test utilization [see comments]. *Clin Biochem* 29, No. 4:291–299. Comment in *Clin Biochem* 1997; 30, No. 4:361, 363.

Medicare Payment Advisory Commission (MedPAC). March 1999. *Report to the Congress: Medicare Payment Policy*. Washington, DC: MedPAC.

Office of the Inspector General (OIG). June 1995. OEI-05-94-00130. *CLIA's Impact on the Availability of Laboratory Services*. Washington, DC: OIG.

van Walraven, C., and C. D. Naylor. 1998. Do we know what inappropriate laboratory utilization is? A systematic review of laboratory clinical audits [see comments]. *JAMA* 280, No. 6:550–558. Comment in *JAMA* 1998; 280, No. 6:565–566.

6

Alternative Payment Methodologies

INTRODUCTION

In response to the charge to assess alternative payment methodologies, the committee identified a range of options for paying for different types of medical services, using the existing literature and surveys and interviews with selected payers and providers.[1] This broad list of options was clearly too extensive for analysis within the time and resources available. The committee, therefore, narrowed its focus to those methods likely to be most suitable to the particular characteristics of clinical laboratory services. Discussion of alternative methodologies in this chapter is organized around the structure and elements of payment systems considered initially in Chapter 4 and the goals that the committee articulated in Chapter 1.[2]

In the next section, the committee analyzes the major elements of a payment system, discusses the alternatives for structuring each element, and assesses the

---

[1]See Appendix C for a description of the methodology used in the payment survey conducted for the Institute of Medicine (IOM) by CHPS Consulting. Katie Merrell (see footnote 2) collected information during January and February 2000 through interviews with several key informants from the laboratory and insurance industries. Informants were identified through specialty societies and other knowledgeable sources and were assured anonymity.

[2]Very little literature exists on the issues surrounding payment methodologies for clinical laboratory services. This chapter, therefore, draws heavily from the literature on paying for other health services providers, particularly physicians, and on general health services research. Much of the chapter is drawn from a paper commissioned by the IOM for this study by Katie Merrell, Center for Health Administration Studies, University of Chicago.

strengths and weaknesses of these options. The third section discusses other key design issues, such as updating the payment schedule, payment adjustments, and cost sharing by beneficiaries. Finally, the chapter concludes with a discussion of implementation considerations, including the legislative and administrative steps necessary for implementation and the paperwork and financial costs of introducing and using the various options.

The current payment system and its various elements were among the options considered by the committee. Since elements of the current payment methodology are discussed extensively in Chapter 4, they are mentioned only briefly in this chapter. Also, the committee's assessment of the current system, discussed in Chapter 5, is not repeated here, but it did influence the discussion of the advantages and disadvantages of the various alternatives.

ELEMENTS OF A PAYMENT SYSTEM

Type of Payment

The committee recognizes the general advantages of prospective payment and did not examine in depth any retrospective payment methods for clinical laboratory services.

Definition

Payment amounts can be determined on a retrospective or prospective basis.[3] Retrospective payment means that the amount paid is determined by (or based on) what the provider charged or said it cost to provide the service after tests or services had been rendered to beneficiaries. Here providers have no incentive to hold down their charges or costs, and the payer has few mechanisms for controlling expenditures (Sing et al, 1998). In a prospective payment system (PPS), prices are set in advance and are known (or knowable) by all parties before care is provided.

Discussion

Prior to 1984, Medicare paid clinical laboratories on a complicated retrospective system, similar to that used to pay physicians. The reasonableness of the charges was judged based on customary, prevailing, and reasonable criteria. Since the mid-1980s Medicare, as well as virtually all private payers, has moved to using prospective payment systems. The Health Care Financing Administration (HCFA) has paid for inpatient hospital services on a prospective basis since 1983. It recently implemented a prospective payment system for outpatient hospital care and is currently designing a PPS for the remaining specialized hospi-

---

[3]Regardless of how the payment amount is determined, payment is made after the test or service is provided or the capitated period has elapsed and a claim filed.

tals not yet covered by a prospective system. Medicare pays for physicians' services on a prospective basis and for laboratory services, defacto, on a prospective basis.

Comparative Assessment

A retrospective payment system gives providers greater influence over payment rates than they generally have under PPS. In turn, it reduces the payers' ability to constrain expenditure growth. The use of prospective payment leads to more predictable payment levels for payers, patients, and providers and is typically associated with simpler administrative systems. Prospective payment systems also provide an opportunity for the payer to exercise some control over total spending through such mechanisms as constraints on updates and volume adjustments.

Unit of Payment

The committee concludes that the risks of a capitated payment for laboratories outweigh its advantages of administrative simplicity and efficiency and that payment per service or test is preferable.

Definition

The unit of payment for laboratory services can be defined in several ways. It can reflect a single test or service, a group of services, or all potential services used by a beneficiary in a specified period (capitation). Under the current payment per test or service, tests are identified and classified through specific HCFA Common Procedural Coding System (HCPCS) codes, which encompass the American Medical Association's (AMA's) Current Procedural Terminology (CPT). A dollar amount is then set for each coded service. Under a method that groups services for payment purposes, related laboratory services are bundled. For example, panels of automated tests are bundled into groups and a payment amount is set for each group of tests. Under capitated payment, the provider is paid a fixed amount per beneficiary for a list of covered tests that may be medically necessary during a given time period. The payment is provided whether or not beneficiaries use any services.

Discussion

Payment per Test. Each test or service has an assigned CPT code or HCPCS code in the case of Medicare. For most tests and services, it is clear to the laboratory which HCPCS code to use. Multiple testing methodologies for a single analyte or similar methodologies testing different analytes may be represented by a single code number, so assigning an appropriate payment amount can sometimes be problematic.

Payment per Group of Tests. For tests that are routinely and frequently ordered together, bundling them and using panel-level payments can create administrative savings to physicians and the program. If the test can be done on a multichannel analyzer, the laboratory's cost savings from performing all of the tests at once should be reflected in the payment. The payment for automated chemistry panels should be less than the sum of payments for individual tests in the panel because of economies of scale. The appropriate use of panel payments is complicated, in part, because the definitions of panels as well as the rules governing their payment have changed frequently over the years. Relatively few tests are included in panel fees, but they tend to be among those most frequently ordered. Grouped or panel tests could be a component of a system using payment per test or service, but could not be a separate option, because bundling is not appropriate for all tests.

Capitation. The use of capitation in the health sector grew during the 1990s. Increasingly, private health plans that receive capitation payments from Medicare under Medicare+Choice or from private purchasers, use capitation payments to buy laboratory services. Two basic approaches are used to capitate laboratories: (1) a managed care organization pays the laboratory an agreed-upon amount per member per month to provide all, or a defined list of, ordered laboratory services; or (2) the managed care organization includes laboratory services in the capitated payment to the physician.[4] The latter approach is rarely used.

Capitated payments for laboratory services under fee-for-service Medicare are conceivable, although the committee is not aware of this method being used. This approach would require Medicare to contract selectively with certain laboratories to provide services to identifiable subgroups of beneficiaries, possibly on the basis of geography. It would be necessary to determine an appropriate per-person capitation payment rate. One or more laboratories would be paid a capitated amount to provide required laboratory services to the covered group of beneficiaries. By determining the size of the covered groups, Medicare would effectively be deciding how many laboratories in each area (or nationwide) would get Medicare business, which in turn could have tremendous implications for the numbers and types of laboratories that survive in future years. Physicians

---

[4]A related payment option would be to integrate Medicare laboratory payments into the fee schedule for physicians providing care under fee for service, not managed care. This would put the physician in control of laboratory test payments as well as ordering. Conceptually, it is closer to a bundled payment than capitation, since payment would be based on a fee for a physician's service, but the physician would be at risk for utilization of laboratory services. Although this approach has been discussed over the years at the theoretical level, practical issues of how to estimate appropriate laboratory payments for each relevant physician service, how to handle variations in testing patterns among specialties, and how to protect the chronically ill from underservice would have to be resolved.

treating beneficiaries and ordering outpatient laboratory tests would have to send patients or specimens to the appropriate selected laboratory, much as they would for private patients in managed care.

Comparative Assessment

Selection of the unit of payment should include consideration of administrative feasibility, efficiency, incentives for appropriate use of services, and adaptability to new technology. The incorporation of new technology into the system is affected by how finely the unit is defined. If the unit were defined by very specific test characteristics, then new service codes and payments would be needed every time a new, slightly different test is approved for Medicare coverage. Conversely, if the unit were defined by broad categories of tests or some basic equivalent service, then new codes and amounts would be needed only for breakthrough technologies that create a new class of test. The gain in administrative simplicity with broad code categories could limit access to new technologies that are not substantially less expensive than existing tests. That situation would arise because manufacturers might be reluctant to develop a new, relatively expensive technology of higher quality that is similar to an existing test and would be included in a current code and payment amount, if they felt the existing fee was insufficient. On the other hand, such a deterrent might be useful in the case of new, more expensive technologies that are not a significant improvement over current methods.

Continued use of payment per test or per service would be most consistent with other Medicare Part B, fee-for-service policies. The current system of payment per service is familiar to all stakeholders, would require no major system change, and could provide a fairer basis for payment than capitation. There would be no disruption to the structure of the laboratory industry with this option. It would be difficult to set an appropriate formula for calculating capitation rates, given the current level of knowledge about clinical laboratory utilization rates by the Medicare population. With test claims data, HCFA could more readily track patterns of practice and costs per episode if it so chose. Because of shortcomings of the current coding system, it would be worthwhile to explore alternatives for future use.

Capitation generally is thought to promote more efficient, appropriate, simple, and financially sustainable care. It also carries the risk of providers' inappropriately using lower-quality tests that are less costly and limiting the number of tests ordered so as not to exceed the constraints of the per capita payment. Because several hundred million outpatient clinical laboratory tests are processed annually by Medicare, using a monthly capitation payment for each participating laboratory would mean a significant reduction in HCFA's administrative burden and costs. It would be an administrative challenge for physicians as well as HCFA, however, to ensure that physicians and patients use the appropriate, capitated laboratories.

With a capitated Medicare laboratory payment, as with capitated laboratory services offered to managed care patients, the laboratory would have no control over utilization. In this situation, the purchaser, Medicare, would also have little control over a physician's test-ordering behavior. Care would not be managed, merely capitated.

The potential effects on the industry of selective contracting for laboratory services would be a drawback of capitation. The possible disruption of the entire structure of the industry under a capitated laboratory payment with very limited numbers of contractors could have a negative impact on beneficiary access, quality, and value. Efforts to mitigate negative effects on the clinical laboratory industry's composition, such as increasing the number of contracted laboratories or frequently revisiting contracts to encourage losers to re-compete and winners to provide good service, would likely increase the administrative complexity of this approach and reduce some of the expected gains.

Basis of Payment

The committee recognizes the advantages of a single, national fee schedule based on resource costs for fee-for-service payment.

Definition

Prospective fee-for-service payment, almost by definition, uses a fee schedule. The question is whether the fee schedule should reflect charges, competitive market prices, favorable pricing, or resource costs. Each option implies a different choice of payment methodology: charge-based payment, competitive bidding, a "most-favored-nation" (MFN) approach, or a fee schedule based on the National Limitation Amounts (NLAs) or resource costs. Some options more naturally lead to multiple fee schedules, while others result in a single national fee schedule. Multiple fee schedules may better reflect local market conditions. A single national fee schedule, however, has the potential to be simpler to administer, more understandable to stakeholders, and more equitable among laboratory service providers.

Discussion

The following sections review two market-oriented approaches for developing fee schedules—competitive bidding and MFN—and two administrative approaches—NLAs and the establishment of a resource-based relative value scale (RBRVS). It is beyond the scope of this study to examine possible barriers to market entry, collusion, or other potential sources of market power in the laboratory testing industry. In addition, the limited availability of information about the current structure, competitiveness, and quality of the laboratory industry makes it impossible for the committee to assess the likely market implications of particular payment approaches. In the following discussion of alternative approaches, there are no precise estimates of how alternative approaches would affect the number and types of laboratories in a particular market. Because current Medicare payment for laboratory services derives from charges and Chapter 5 has assessed the merits of this charge-based payment, using charges as the basis of payment is not reviewed in this chapter outside the discussion of the NLA.

Competitive Bidding. This is a method by which buyers and sellers come to agree on prices. Competition among sellers to win business encourages each to reveal the minimum price at which a sale is acceptable. The goal of competitive bidding is to secure for Medicare a set of prices that reflect the cost of efficient production, including a normal profit. Bidding is supposed to discover these prices without the need for intrusive data collection or any explicit decision by Medicare about the amount of profit to be earned by individual firms.

The key to competitive bidding as a strategy for developing appropriate rates is in how the auction is actually structured. There are several design issues discussed below that could affect the operation of competitive bidding as well as the results.[5] For purchasing clinical laboratory services, HCFA has developed various competitive bidding models that typically have the following features:

1. Multiple contracts would be awarded to avoid the risk of bad performance. This would allow physicians and their patients to move their business to laboratories that give satisfactory quality and service.
2. Laboratories would bid a price for each of a set of tests. These bids would typically be weighted by volume and evaluated. Winners would be selected based on a stated protocol. They would receive no guarantee of business, only a right to market their services and be paid at the winning prices. The number of winners would affect the number of fee schedules in use.
3. Bidders whose prices were too high either would be excluded from participating in the demonstration area during the period of the demonstration or would be allowed to participate at a discounted rate. Exclusion of losers would enhance the value of being a winner by increasing the prospect of business.
4. In most designs, bids would be required from all commercial laboratories and from hospitals that market outpatient laboratory services to the general population of physicians. Physician office laboratories (POLs) would not be required to bid and would automatically be paid at the winning prices. If there were federal budget constraints on Medicare, an upper limit on the bidding process might be necessary.

---

[5]An extensive economics literature on the nature of auctions provides insights into how to structure the bidding process to minimize gaming and yield bids that are likely to reflect efficiency prices. Mennemeyer (1989, pp. 326–331), discusses some of these issues with regard to laboratory services; McAfee and McMillan (1987) provide a general overview of auctions and how their structure affects resulting prices.

5. Prices determined by competitive bidding would be exempt from federal budget adjustments or rate cuts during the period of the procurement. Price updates would occur automatically with each round of competitive bidding procurement.

Strengths of Competitive Bidding. Competitive bidding should produce prices that are close to bidders' actual costs. Conventional economic analysis, if applied to this issue, would suggest that competitive bidding could encourage lower costs and innovation by limiting existing firms' market power. The government expects that these prices would, in most cases, be lower than those it pays under the current laboratory fee schedule and thus produce a net savings in total expenditures for Medicare, but this is not certain. There would be minimal disclosure of business data since laboratories would not have to reveal the basis for their bid, the details of their cost structure, or the amount of their profit.

HCFA became interested in competitive bidding for outpatient clinical laboratory services in the mid-1980s and issued contracts for both sizable studies of the laboratory industry and design options for a demonstration. Since 1995, HCFA has invested more than $350,000 and has created a significant body of literature analyzing design alternatives for competitive bidding (Hoerger and Waters, 1993; Hoerger et al., 1997; Mennemeyer et al., 1986). HCFA has an operational demonstration in one county for competitive bidding on durable medical equipment and supplies and it resulted in first-year aggregate savings of 17 percent, without a reduction in access. (DeParle and Berenson, 2000).

Weaknesses of Competitive Bidding. Under an exclusive bidding model, or selective contracting, where only firms submitting winning bids would be allowed to participate in Medicare, losing firms would not be able to participate in the Medicare program in the designated area during the time of the procurement. This could have a significant effect on the financial health of excluded laboratories and the structure of the entire industry. Even without the exclusion of losers, the impact of competitive bidding could disproportionately disadvantage certain segments of the laboratory industry. The committee had insufficient data to conclude whether the present number and mix of laboratories is appropriate or not to meet Medicare beneficiaries' needs most efficiently. Hence it makes no recommendation whether the current size and structure of the laboratory industry should be maintained or changed. Nevertheless, the committee recognizes that policy changes that do significantly change the structure of the industry would likely have more short-run implications for Medicare beneficiaries and physicians than would policies that maintain the status quo. Such changes may be appropriate and desirable, but it is important that they be anticipated and steps taken to minimize the dislocations experienced by beneficiaries as they occur. The committee thought there might be efficiency gains from competitive bidding in terms of Medicare payments for services in some markets, but it is unclear how they would compare with the added administrative costs of running competitive bidding processes. Hence, a demonstration would provide useful experience and data.

Competitive bidding would likely result in multiple fee schedules across the country and possibly even within separate bidding areas. This could add administrative complexities to the program and has the potential for laboratories in different areas to be treated unequally.

The committee believes that developing a feasible competitive bidding process requires testing through a demonstration in order to gather information about the needs for administrative resources, HCFA management at the local level, how beneficiaries and physicians would respond, how to educate them, and how their access to services would be affected. Although much developmental work has already been done, it would nevertheless take an extended time for a demonstration to become operational and evaluation findings to be available. At that point, it should be clearer whether the approach would be practical and advantageous on a national or local level.

There has been much opposition from the laboratory industry to competitive bidding. HCFA's work was halted in 1987 when Congress imposed a moratorium in response to industry opposition. Provider opposition has prevented implementation of all Medicare competitive bidding demonstrations other than the one for durable medical equipment, not just the ones for laboratories. A former HCFA administrator concluded recently that the failure of competitive pricing demonstrations four times, in part due to the lack of broad political support, did not bode well for HCFA to develop new market-based approaches for Medicare (DeParle and Berenson, 2000).

The committee finds that the disadvantages of competitive bidding outweigh its advantages for use as the basis of payment. Nevertheless, it considers this method again as a possible means of collecting data that could inform calculation of the level of payment.

Most-Favored-Nation Approach. This title is borrowed from the language of international trade and refers to a system in which laboratories would provide services to Medicare beneficiaries for the lowest rate they accept from any other payer. In effect, each laboratory would create its own Medicare fee schedule. This approach would tend to eliminate laboratory discounts to selected private payers. In theory, the MFN approach could lead to economically efficient pricing across payers, minimizing the risk of Medicare subsidizing the discount that laboratories offer to other payers. It is uncertain how laboratories would translate private capitation rates into reasonably comparable amounts or fees per individual tests. Even comparisons of Medicare test fees with those of private payers can be difficult if the private payer includes different bundles of tests in its panels. MFN would result in variation among laboratories in relative and actual payment rates. It is not clear what enforcement policies, such as audits and reporting requirements, would be necessary to ensure that providers charge Medicare no more than their lowest commercial rate.

A concern of some laboratorians is that, although the test may be the same, services provided to Medicare are not comparable to the services that laboratories offer other payers because the laboratory must provide substantially more documentation for Medicare. Thus, the costs of doing business with Medicare may exceed the costs of serving private patients. Some laboratories feel justified in charging Medicare more to cover these costs. The committee has found no cost data to support or refute this claim.

Strengths of MFN. In theory, the MFN approach would allow Medicare to pay no more than private payers and could create a more equitable arrangement among all payers. It would not initially require extensive and possibly intrusive data collection. To the extent that Medicare has been cross-subsidizing lower rates to physicians or other private payers, this approach could produce lower payments for Medicare.

Weaknesses of MFN. The biggest drawback of MFN is the difficulty in ensuring that laboratories charge Medicare according to the rules. Detection and prevention of fraud could present major administrative problems. Other administrative functions, such as changes in computer systems to accommodate laboratory-specific fees that change continually could also cause difficulties. The MFN system could become costly if laboratories were less willing to bargain for discounted rates with managed care companies because the same rates apply to Medicare. If Medicaid was the lowest payer in a market, however, the laboratories probably would not have the same flexibility to negotiate rates with the state as they do with private payers. If Medicaid was included in the MFN approach, it could significantly lower Medicare rates for laboratories in these states or create an incentive for laboratories to drop out of the Medicaid program. Substantial developmental work would be necessary to design an MFN system, and as with competitive bidding, demonstrations would be desirable before national implementation is considered.

National Limitation Amounts. Initially, HCFA could consider establishing a single national fee schedule based on NLAs. This would look very much like current payments since most of the fees and even more of the payments (98 percent) are now constrained by the NLAs (Appendix B).

Strengths of NLAs. NLAs are available, known to all stakeholders, would cause minimal disruption to the industry, and would likely have a negligible effect on beneficiary access in the short-term. Since these fees are within the range of private payer fees, NLAs have face validity. A single, national fee schedule would be simpler to manage and explain to stakeholders than multiple fee schedules such as the current 56 carrier fee schedules or laboratory-specific schedules.

Weaknesses of NLAs. NLAs are based on historical charges, which may bear little logical relationship to the costs of providing specific laboratory services now. If used indefinitely, they could distort incentives for laboratories to offer certain tests.

Resource-Based Relative Value Scale. HCFA spent millions of dollars during the late 1980s and 1990s to develop an RBRVS for physician services. Much of the theoretical and practical lessons from that experience could inform the development of a resource-based fee schedule for clinical laboratory tests or services. Such a relative value scale (RVS) requires data on actual or estimated resources used for individual laboratory tests or services and shows the relative relationship of these resources from one test to another. Methods for collecting the necessary data on resources, including costs for equipment, supplies, labor, and other direct and indirect costs, used to produce laboratory services and their cost are discussed in the next section. The relationship of payments across services affects providers' relative willingness to provide each service and in turn can affect efficiency, appropriateness, technological innovation, access, and the composition of the industry.

Policymakers have to consider whether such a relative value scale should be based on the costs or resources of an efficient laboratory (and how such a laboratory would be defined and identified), on the mean or median costs or resources of all laboratories (or a sample), or on some other measure. These design decisions will be important to stakeholders and will affect the way relative values are developed and the cost of their development, but it is not clear how much impact such a decision would have on relative, rather than actual, levels of payment. For example, the actual dollar cost of a test in an efficient laboratory might be significantly lower than the mean or median cost of all laboratories. Nonetheless, the cost of Test A might be twice as much as that of Test B, whether it was conducted in an efficient laboratory or a laboratory with median costs. The relative values would be the same in the different laboratories, although the level of costs would differ.

Strengths of an RBRVS. Relative values based on costs or resources would likely minimize financial distortions or incentives to provide some services rather than others (PPRC, 1989). In any case, the creation of some cost or resource-based data on laboratory tests is essential to assessing the adequacy of current and future payment levels. It would not be necessary to have precise data on each of the 1,100 codes in order to establish a laboratory RBRVS. Data on some tests within groups of closely related codes could be used to estimate values for those codes lacking data. Such a scale could readily be converted to dollar amounts for a single national fee schedule by the use of a dollar conversion factor and adjusted as necessary.

Weaknesses of an RBRVS. A relative value approach could be very difficult to design because the resource costs are difficult to establish. Furthermore, some frequently performed tests or services are parts of panels that use the same specimen and equipment for all tests. The costs associated with each test are almost impossible to separate accurately. Also, there are numerous challenges to collecting cost data from laboratories.

Level of Payment

If a resource-based relative value scale were used to determine payments for clinical laboratory services, multiple approaches could contribute useful information on resource costs for developing the relative value scale. Issues related to setting the initial conversion factor also must be addressed.

Definition

A fee schedule shows the payment amount set for each test or service—that is, the level of payment. The previous discussion on the basis of payment noted that certain payment methods would automatically result in a dollar payment level: competitive bidding, MFN, and the NLA. The RBRVS would result in a list of ratios showing the relationship of each test to a standard test. A conversion factor would have to be used to turn ratios reflecting the relative value of each test into dollars.[6]

Discussion

This subsection reviews four approaches that the committee considered for collecting the data necessary to establish resource-based relative values. If it were possible to collect consistent, accurate cost data readily from a sufficiently large sample of laboratories for each test on the fee schedule, this discussion would be simpler, but obtaining objective and reliable data is difficult. Each approach to developing a laboratory RBRVS has its own strengths and limitations. The approaches differ with regard to cost and likely acceptance by stakeholders. Some of these approaches may be more easily adapted than others to setting national relative values. They are not mutually exclusive, and by using an appropriate combination of approaches, perhaps the weaknesses of each can be minimized. The options include micro-costing studies, a consensus approach, charges, and demonstrations using competitive bidding or negotiations.

Regardless of the approach adopted to establish relative values, a resource-based fee schedule also needs a dollar conversion factor to translate the RVS into payment amounts. This combination of the RVS and the conversion factor determines the fee schedule's level of payments. Setting the initial conversion

---

[6]If the relative values were based directly on dollar fees, the conversion factor would, in effect, be 1.0.

factor for a newly established fee schedule is thus a critical policy decision. Considerations in setting the conversion factor are discussed at the close of this subsection.

Micro-Costing Studies. Micro-costing studies using standard accounting practices involve collecting detailed data on direct costs and developing an appropriate basis for allocating indirect costs to specific services to create service-level cost estimates. Direct costs are those that are incurred in providing a specific service to a particular patient; indirect costs are those that would accrue regardless of the number or mix of services provided in a particular day. The lack of standard cost accounting systems for the laboratory's costs, distinct and separate from the hospital or physician's practice makes any data collection difficult. In addition, there are no consensus documents or conventional methods for micro-cost accounting that are agreed on by laboratory experts and used throughout the industry. To reduce problems of comparability of data from laboratory to laboratory, any cost study would have to establish definitions that are meaningful to survey respondents, regardless of their own accounting practices. There also has to be a standardized method to allocate indirect costs that is used consistently from laboratory to laboratory.

Collecting data on direct costs is a serious challenge in micro-costing studies. A number of important methodological issues have to be addressed that will affect the quality and collection costs of the data and stakeholder acceptance of both the process and the outcome. Decisions must be made about the type of sample: Should it be representative of all laboratories, of laboratories weighted by Medicare service volume or revenue, of "efficient" laboratories, or of some other group of laboratories? Similarly, the question of how to administer the survey and validate results—by phone, by mail, or in person—also has important implications for data costs and validity.

Strengths of Micro-Costing Studies. The cost data acquisition method not only is important for establishing initial relative values, but also could be used on a periodic basis for contributing to reviews of the relative values. It also could provide insight into whether Medicare was paying the "right price" for a particular test. The size of the sample, number of tests, and specific research methods could be scaled according to the research funds available.

Weaknesses of Micro-Costing Studies. Such an approach has been used in limited ways to date, but it has not yet been used successfully on a national basis to establish national Medicare payment rates for any providers. HCFA incorporated a modest, reasonably simple, cost survey administered by mail, with phone follow-up, as part of its efforts to develop new practice expense relative values for the Medicare Fee Schedule for physicians. HCFA discontinued the survey because of the low response rate of less than 30 percent to the first round of the study.

The committee used a very small resource-costing study to gain insight into how current payment rates relate to service-level costs and to understand the process that would be required to conduct such a study on a broader scale.[7] The cost survey, including site visits, encountered serious difficulties. Researchers found no uniformity of existing accounting systems from laboratory to laboratory and a reluctance of laboratories to participate in a time-consuming data collection process without compensation. Given the current sensitivity of the laboratory industry to divulging cost data, the potential response to a HCFA cost survey could be poor if there were no direct incentives or penalties associated with responding.

Consensus Approach. A consensus approach relies on interdisciplinary groups of experts and aims to get some estimate of relative costs or resource use at the service or test level. It can be structured to provide opportunities for public input. Because this approach is used to develop relative values, not to set prices, it can minimize the potential for anti-competitive regulatory capture. Data-driven consensus approaches can have more credibility and can lead to more accurate results than micro-costing studies alone. Data drawn from various sources—including audits, competitive bidding and negotiations, and actual costs and charges—can inform, challenge, and validate the decisions of a consensus panel.

This approach has been used to establish physician work and practice expense values under the physician fee schedule and is the basis for periodic review of the entire fee schedule. As a result, HCFA has experience in establishing this type of process, working with providers, and using the results to develop (and later refine) relative values.

Strengths of the Consensus Approach. This approach could be much less expensive than an extensive micro-costing effort. It could be readily used in conjunction with other approaches to integrate data from various sources. If well structured, it can enhance the credibility of the resulting relative values among stakeholders.

Weaknesses of the Consensus Approach. Considerable attention must be given to structuring the process because the acceptability of the results to stakeholders will likely depend largely on their view of the fairness of the process used to select participants, the structure of the meetings, and how rigorously

---

[7]CHPS Consulting, which conducted the study, used *resource costing,* a methodology for gathering cost data when the data are not readily available through conventional accounting systems. Activities are broken down into discrete components, and the resources for each component are identified. The quantity of each resource used is measured, and a unit price for the resource is obtained. Once these data are available, the cost for each resource can be calculated. The sum of the costs of each resource is the cost of the activity.

information is used to establish relative values. Care must be taken to avoid the possibility or appearance of regulatory capture.

Charges. Relative charges could be accepted as a reasonable indicator of relative costs, could be compared with cost data to establish the relationship initially, or could provide the starting point for a consensus process. Since charge data are continuously updated and available to HCFA, they could also be used for future revisions of the national fee schedule.

Strengths of Charges. Developing charge-based relative values would be relatively inexpensive and administratively simple since HCFA has charges recorded on all laboratory claims submitted for payment. In addition, a charge-based system provides an automatic and timely methodology for accommodating the need to set payments for new laboratory tests and for updating the relative values of the national fee schedule.

Weaknesses of Charges. This approach is based on the assumption that charges are highly correlated with costs. That assumption may be spurious, and any correlation may vary for different types of providers and different markets, and be affected by payment policies of major payers. Without reasonable evidence that charges accurately reflect costs, stakeholders unhappy with the approach could present data showing low correlation between charges and costs, undermining the credibility of the new fee schedule.

Competitive Bidding and Negotiation Demonstrations. Information on relative prices resulting from a competitive bidding demonstration could provide the basis for setting relative values. The demonstration could be structured to provide data for establishing initial relative values and would not necessarily be repeated annually or implemented in a manner that ultimately excluded laboratories in the demonstration sites. Although the resulting prices from this competitive bidding demonstration would be used only to establish relative values, not actual payment rates, they could provide information for assessing whether Medicare is paying too little for laboratory services or is a relatively generous payer.

A variant of competitive bidding would be a demonstration using a negotiation process to establish acceptable fees that could be the basis for calculating relative values. This approach would draw from experience in the private sector, since some health plans negotiate contracts directly with laboratories. For Medicare, the carrier could negotiate with laboratories in its area.

Strengths of Competitive Bidding and Negotiation Demonstrations. These approaches could reveal market prices and the relationship between payments for one test and another with minimal federal intrusion. HCFA has done considerable research on competitive bidding. On a demonstration basis, these approaches would not be as disruptive to the industry or as expensive to implement as they could be on a national basis.

Weaknesses of Competitive Bidding and Negotiation Demonstrations. There might be distortions from using data from a few demonstration sites to set national relative values. Laboratories might not be interested in bidding or negotiating if the outcome was to be used primarily for calculating national relative values, not their own payment rates. The negotiating capability of small laboratories, especially POLs, could bias the results, since POLs probably have had relatively little experience negotiating payment rates with health plans. Negotiations with the large number of POLs could also be an overwhelming administrative burden for the carrier.

Setting the Initial Conversion Factor. Once the RVS is established, the conversion factor that translates relative values into payment amounts must be set. The level of the conversion factor has implications for all stakeholders. From the Medicare program's perspective, the lowest conversion factor that will not compromise beneficiary access both reflects prudent purchasing and contributes to the longer-term financial sustainability of the program. Because it is difficult to determine precisely what that conversion factor would be, there is a risk of setting payment rates too low, which would make serving Medicare beneficiaries less attractive and less feasible for the laboratories. The information on costs and prices collected while developing the relative value scale could provide some indication of the adequacy of payment rates and guidance in setting the conversion factor. At the same time, the parameters for setting the initial conversion factor are likely to be specified by the Congress. Under current budget and legislative requirements, Congress may mandate that implementation of a new fee schedule for clinical laboratory services not increase program spending. Maintaining budget neutrality—ensuring the same level of spending for laboratory services under the new system as would have occurred under the system it replaced—would impose constraints on the level of the initial conversion factor.

OTHER ISSUES IN PAYMENT SYSTEMS

Updating Payments

The committee recognizes that both the mechanism used and the factors to be considered in keeping a laboratory fee schedule up to date will depend on the basis of payment chosen and the method used to determine payment levels.

How payment systems change over time depends on a number of factors. Retrospective payment systems, such as cost-based and charge-based systems, are self-updating: as costs or charges increase, so do payment rates. This is exactly the characteristic of prior payment systems that led payers, including Medicare, to adopt administratively set updates that adjust for expected or desirable changes over time while providing some control over spending growth. For some prospective payment systems, the method of determining payments also automatically changes them over time. For example, MFN fee schedules for laboratory services would unilaterally be updated continuously for each laboratory, and payments under a competitive bidding methodology would be updated with each bidding cycle. In all of these cases, the payment changes that would naturally occur could be constrained by congressional action if the Congress were to choose to control spending. For example, the NLAs currently constrain the extent to which changes in charges will be reflected in Medicare payments. In a similar manner, Congress could set an upper bound for payments determined through competitive bidding. Prior to the Medicare Fee Schedule, updates in Medicare's charge-based payments were constrained by the Medicare Economic Index.

Total program spending is determined by both payment levels and service volumes, and payers can consider the relation between the two when they set annual updates. These administratively determined updates, which are increasingly common among payers, take into account factors such as input price inflation and expected service volume and intensity changes due to changes in technology, the demographics of the enrolled population, and services covered, or shifts in services that are complements or substitutes for those in another service sector.

Medicare has adopted an approach to updating the conversion factor for the physician fee schedule that results in lower updates when volume growth exceeds expectations and higher updates when volume growth is less than expected. This method is designed to hold total spending to anticipated targets. The update mechanism includes laboratory service volume in the annual measure of volume used to set future physician payment updates. Thus, excessive growth in laboratory spending could negatively affect future physician fees. Laboratory services are provided on referral from physicians. For this reason, laboratory volume growth is, to a large extent, beyond the control of laboratories. Placing the responsibility for laboratory volume growth on physicians, by considering laboratory service volume in physician fee updates, is likely to be more effective than having a separate volume target for updating laboratory fees. Adjustments for input price growth for laboratory services, however, would still be necessary.

Keeping a payment system current depends on more than annual fee updates. It requires periodic review and revision of all key policy elements, because the way in which services are produced and used changes over time. Different payment methods will pose different administrative challenges related to the way they are structured. For example, the relative values in the Medicare Fee Schedule for physicians are now subject to review every five years by AMA's RVS Update Committee (RUC) and HCFA.[8] This provides an opportunity to

---

[8]Initial implementation of the fee schedule required refinement of newly established relative values. Once this refinement process was complete, the RVS became subject to review every five years. (See PPRC, 1995, pp. 39–41, for an assessment of the RUC and

ensure that annual additions of new services to the RVS and other refinements to specific relative values do not lead to distortions in the relative value scale over time.

Adjustments

The committee has found no evidence to suggest that there are currently beneficiary access problems or other concerns that would need correcting through an adjustment to the laboratory fee schedule. If a new payment system were adopted, there could be a need for certain payment adjustments depending on how the method is structured. Examination of the appropriateness and implications of making adjustments for factors such as geographic cost differences, sole community hospital costs, access in rural areas, or STAT tests thus follows decisions about the payment method.

Because circumstances change over time, monitoring the impact of the payment system, and any modifications to it, on beneficiary access, laboratory participation, and program costs may identify areas in which future adjustments would be appropriate. The current system, based on 56 locally set fee schedules, conceptually includes a geographic adjustment, although geographic variations in payments are limited by the NLA. It also includes an adjustment for sole community hospitals. The appropriateness of these and other adjustments depends on whether the current system remains unchanged or the committee's recommendations are implemented.

Some of the committee's stated goals could be achieved through explicit adjustments made to payments, depending on the design of key elements of the payment system. For example, under a national fee schedule, payments could be adjusted for local differences in costs in order to promote provider equity. Such an adjustment would require decisions about the geographic units within which laboratory payments would be equal and about the most suitable price index or indices to use for adjusting payments. The Medicare Fee Schedule for physicians and the hospital inpatient PPS provide different models for approaching these decisions.[9]

Special adjusters could also explicitly promote the goal of patient access if instances of precarious or inappropriately limited access could be objectively identified. For example, Medicare physician payments are increased for care provided to beneficiaries who live in health professional shortage areas (HPSAs), in an effort to improve access to physician services for beneficiaries in these areas, Omnibus Budget Reconciliation Act (OBRA, 1989). Any evidence that labora-

---

the first five-year review process and pp. 50–51 for a discussion of other issues that may be relevant to periodic review.)

[9]See Committee on Ways and Means, (1998, pp. 1118–1125, 1195–1198) for details about geographic adjustment of hospital and physician payments, respectively.

tory services are unavailable in particular communities could support some comparable adjustments to help promote the development of a local service supply.

Specific adjustments based on site of service have been proposed for laboratory payments. Underlying the use of adjusted payments in different settings is the notion that unit costs differ for different types or settings of laboratories and that the lack of such a site adjustment would make it difficult for settings with higher costs to continue to provide services. Opponents of such adjustments argue that there is no reason for Medicare to pay more for services in the higher-cost setting if they are available for less in other settings.

Under current policy, laboratories in qualified sole community hospitals are paid slightly more. The committee found no data with which to determine whether sole community hospitals, in fact, do have higher laboratory costs, the current adjustment is an appropriate amount, or there would be access problems for beneficiaries if the adjustment was eliminated. Likewise, the committee found neither cost data nor evidence on access to support the need for an adjustment for other types of laboratory settings, such as hospital-based laboratories or POLs.

There may be some service characteristics for which higher payments are justified. For example, some assert that hospital laboratories incur higher costs because of their need to have equipment available to provide services on an emergency, or STAT, basis.[10] In this case, it may be appropriate to have a payment adjustment for STAT services, regardless of site, if providing quick turnaround is typically associated with higher costs and is viewed as clinically important in some circumstances.

The risk of a STAT adjuster is upcoding—creating an increase in the number of laboratory services performed on a STAT basis in order to bill at the higher amount if this would increase profits. The fact that the physician, not the laboratory, orders tests could limit opportunities for upcoding. Successful implementation of a STAT adjuster, however, would require carefully crafted descriptions of the circumstances under which STAT services are viewed as appropriate. Close monitoring of the medical necessity of these claims might be necessary.

Cost Sharing

The committee concludes that because of the administrative costs and burdens it would impose and the limited effect it would have on reducing excess testing, cost sharing for laboratory services is inconsistent with its goals for a laboratory payment system that ensures beneficiary access and maintains administrative simplicity.

---

[10]This point was made by several speakers at the Institute of Medicine's January 20, 2000, meeting. See, for example, the testimony of the College of American Pathologists (Raslavicus, January 20, 2000).

Payers often use cost sharing to reduce overutilization of insured services. There is evidence of general overuse of health services in the United States, and laboratory services are not an exception to this pattern (Axt-Adam et al., 1993; Hindmarsh and Lyon, 1996; van Walraven and Naylor, 1998).

Currently there is no cost sharing associated with laboratory services used by Medicare beneficiaries, although there was under the charge-based payment system used in the early years of Medicare.[11] Two different justifications have been offered for the present lack of beneficiary cost sharing for laboratory services.[12] First, the referral nature of these services diminishes the potential for inappropriate patient overuse that is typically assumed in cases where services are fully paid by insurance. The lack of cost sharing for laboratory services presumably creates fewer additional program costs than it would for services that are fully covered by insurance and are sought directly by patients. Second, the relatively low levels of payment for many common laboratory services have led many observers to claim that the cost to laboratories of collecting the standard 20 percent copayment amount from beneficiaries would frequently outweigh the revenue generated. In fact, it is estimated that a 20 percent copayment would average less than $2.30 per test for the top 100 laboratory procedures, according to HCFA data.

Despite these arguments, the President's originally submitted FY 2001 budget included a 20 percent copayment for clinical laboratory services meant to prevent overuse and reduce fraud (President's FY 2001 Budget Proposal, 2000). However, HCFA actuaries did not expect the proposal to have a significant impact on utilization.[13]

Options to avoid the impracticalities of collecting copayments for relatively inexpensive services have been proposed but found lacking. One suggestion was the introduction of copayments only for services (individual or total ordered) with payments above some dollar threshold amount. Alternatively a copayment could be applied only for tests at sites where the beneficiary has direct contact with the laboratory and the provider could collect the copayment at the time of testing. These might include POLs, hospital-based laboratories, or independent laboratory specimen collection stations. Each of these options raises issues of administrative complexity, inequitable application of cost sharing, burden on the laboratories, and potential ineffectiveness in reducing unnecessary utilization.

---

[11]The cost-sharing requirement for laboratory services was removed in 1984 as part of a compromise that required laboratories to accept assignment, direct billing, and the imposition of fee schedules set at 60 percent of the prevailing charge.

[12]Both issues were raised in testimony to the committee. See, for example, the statement of the American Association for Clinical Chemistry (Root, January 20, 2000).

[13]The Congressional Budget Office (CBO) also discussed a cost-sharing option that would include a 20 percent copayment plus application of the Part B deductible to laboratory services. The CBO proposal includes use of a deductible as well as a copayment and projects savings of $5.1 billion over five years, most of which again are attributed to factors other than stimulating more appropriate use of laboratory services (CBO, 2000).

Any expected revenue gains from new cost-sharing requirements therefore have to be weighed against the potential costs to laboratories of implementing them, the access barriers that they could present for some beneficiaries, and the potential equity issues raised at the beneficiary and provider levels.

Some cost-sharing alternatives would shift the collection burden from laboratories to other parties. For example, one way to reduce the administrative costs to laboratories of a cost-sharing requirement would be to have the referring physician collect it from the beneficiary along with the copayment for associated physician services. Physicians, however, are likely to resist taking on this role. It is unclear how they would know the appropriate amount to charge the beneficiary. Another way to shift some of the administrative burden associated with cost sharing away from laboratories would be through the introduction of a deductible that was administered by HCFA and the carriers.

Advantages of Beneficiary Cost Sharing. Beneficiary cost sharing for laboratory services will produce savings for Medicare. The administration's budget estimates substantial savings to Medicare of $2.4 billion over the next five years, primarily from the reduction of Medicare spending from 100 percent to 80 percent of the fees. Under the alternative where the physician initially pays the copayment to the laboratory, introducing the beneficiary's costs into the physician–beneficiary relationship might help make both more aware of the costs of laboratory services and less likely to use unnecessary services, restoring some of the educational role of cost sharing into the overall demand for insured services.

Disadvantages of Beneficiary Cost Sharing. Although the rationale given for the cost-sharing budget proposal is to prevent overuse of services, this is not the expectation. In fact, the expected savings would come mainly from shifting costs from Medicare to beneficiaries and laboratories, not from more appropriate use of laboratory services that would produce real savings for the health care system. Instituting any form of cost sharing could create access problems, at least for some beneficiaries (Solanki and Schauffler, 1999; Solanki et al., 2000). Many beneficiaries have some form of supplemental insurance that likely would cover the costs of their laboratory copayments. Those who do not have supplemental insurance, however, are among the most vulnerable elderly and would be the most adversely affected. Evidence suggests that low-income individuals react to cost sharing through decreased use of all services, not just those of limited health value (Brook et al., 1984). These same access problems are associated with all cost-sharing requirements in Medicare.

Cost sharing would also introduce new administrative burdens to the system, whether borne by laboratories, referring physicians, beneficiaries, or Medicare. It could also increase costs to laboratories or referring physicians due to bad debt and to beneficiaries who currently do not pay cost sharing for laboratory services. Having the physician collect the copayment would add significant complexity to the system. The expectation that beneficiaries would become more aware of fraudulent practices because of their copayments seems unrealistic, since they generally are not familiar with the variety of tests available, the appropriate use of various tests, or even the laboratory to which the physician sends their specimen. Significant fraudulent practices by laboratories are more likely to be detected by whistle-blowers than by beneficiaries.

The copayment alternatives based on a dollar threshold or applied only to providers with direct contact with beneficiaries would raise issues of equity for beneficiaries. Beneficiaries who received testing services from independent laboratories that were exempted from collecting copayments would have a financial advantage over those who had to pay on the spot because they had direct contact with the laboratories that conducted their tests. Applying a dollar threshold for tests before the laboratory copayment could be charged would create an incentive to game the system. Beneficiaries who had multiple services simultaneously could be subjected to cost sharing, while those who were able to receive the same tests on separate occasions might have individual charges that stayed below the cost-sharing threshold.

MAKING IMPROVEMENTS A REALITY

Designing Payment Policies

Any change in payment methods can cause major concerns since the economic well-being of so many players is involved, but the apprehension and disruption accompanying such changes can be minimized. During HCFA's implementation of the Medicare physician fee schedule, observers noted that there were a number of aspects of the design and implementation phase that contributed to an apparently smooth process (Oliver, 1993; Smith, 1992):

- A single, comprehensive proposal for reform was able to provide some elements that were attractive to each constituency, along with less popular policies, by combining several key policy changes into one package.
- A consensus approach, open meetings, constructive engagement with all interested stakeholders, and well-regarded staff analyses contributed to an acceptable reform proposal.

These observations suggest a number of considerations for designing and implementing new payment policies for laboratory services.

Anticipate Effects of New Policies. Before a new approach to paying for laboratory services under fee-for-service Medicare is proposed for legislation and implementation, its potential implications for beneficiaries, providers, and the Medicare program should be carefully assessed. Understanding the potential effects of policy change allows the development of mechanisms to identify important problems that arise as new payments are introduced and to respond promptly to them. Clear, accurate information about likely effects of new rates may also help key actors; even those who may not benefit from them, accept them.

In some alternatives previously discussed, the short-run dislocations might be minimal for laboratory providers. To the extent that laboratories provide a broad array of services at volumes comparable to overall Medicare utilization rates, a decision by Congress to mandate a budget-neutral fee-for-service payment change should not have a significant short-term effect on a laboratory's Medicare revenues unless the laboratory is in a geographic area that would see many of its local fees increased. Also, an increase in some fees and a decrease in others, which could happen with a move to resource-based relative values, would balance out in laboratories with average Medicare utilization of services. Nevertheless, any changes are likely to have some impact on the operations of individual laboratories.

Plan to Minimize Dislocations. Strategies for minimizing potential short-run dislocations caused by new policies could be worthwhile depending on the magnitude of anticipated changes. Payment changes could have more serious effects on individual laboratories or on segments of the industry. If their service mixes were different from the overall Medicare distribution, then some laboratories could realize dramatic revenue increases, while others would experience losses. For example, only laboratories certified as high complexity by the Clinical Laboratory Improvement Amendments (CLIA) can do the full range of tests, and some of those laboratories specialize in only a selected menu. Most POLs do only a very limited range of tests. If information about laboratory-specific service mixes suggests that laboratories with certain service mixes would be disproportionately affected by payment changes, it might be appropriate to phase in new payment rates over several years. This would give laboratories a chance to respond to payment changes through changes in staffing, purchasing, or other appropriate strategies. Identifying ways to reduce the shocks associated with a new payment system becomes more difficult the more the proposed changes differ from the current system. For example, in a payment system based on selective contracting with a limited number of providers, it would be impossible to eliminate the dramatic effect on the composition of the industry.

Plan to Monitor Continuing Effects of Changes. Besides finding ways to help ensure smooth implementation of a new system, plans should be made to monitor the effect of new rates on beneficiary access. The clear difficulty here is that changes in service use from current volumes are not necessarily evidence of problems since there is no way to confirm that the present distribution of laboratory services is optimal. As new policies are crafted and proposed, stakeholders will likely present analyses of how payments under the proposed policies will differ in allegedly harmful ways from the current distribution of Medicare laboratory payments. It is difficult to weigh such evidence, however, since it does not clarify the underlying issue of beneficiaries' ability to get needed services on a timely basis under either the current or any proposed system. Knowing that decreased payment for a particular service may reduce its use compared to current rates is not equivalent to knowing that the decreased payment has important implications for beneficiaries' health. Evidence of changes in service use must be combined with other studies that link utilization rates to clinical appropriateness.

Plan for Continuing Operations. Plans should be developed for ongoing administration of the new system. Issues that are important at the time of initial implementation may be quite different from those that require attention once the new system is in place. The methods used to develop initial payment rates may not be the same ones that should be used to update or revise them. Two predictable issues for smooth operation of a new system are its ability (1) to incorporate new technologies and to (2) adjust to changes over time in the costs of providing existing services. Before new payment policies are implemented, attention must be paid to how these longer-run needs will be addressed. Otherwise, the new system would be changed constantly but unpredictably, undermining stakeholders' confidence in it and possibly diminishing the chance that it works as desired or expected.

Implementing New Payment Policies

Implementation of any payment alternatives discussed would depend on many details and design questions to be answered during the planning and development phase for a new methodology. The committee's intent in assessing various payment options and making its recommendations is that any changes made be consistent with the goals of administrative simplicity, efficiency, and transparency. The size and scope of any proposed solutions ought to be reasonably related to the size of the problems.

To discuss legislative amendments, administrative steps, paperwork requirements, and costs for implementation of a payment methodology in any detail, one would have to know very specific aspects of each of the method's elements. Getting data for such a discussion would be sufficiently expensive that it should not be attempted for hypothetical options or general recommendations. More decisions would have to be made and details clarified in order to make realistic assumptions that are needed for cost projections. Hence, the committee decided to discuss implementation issues at a general level and compare options to each other and to the current system. Keep in mind, however, that any change is likely to entail at least some changeover costs, dislocations, and inconveniences, even with careful planning. The alternative of totally maintaining the status quo, with no changes to the current payment methodology, also has costs both for today and, even more, for the future (see Chapter 5 for an assessment of the status quo).

Legislative Changes. Essentially any alternative for payment that would change or eliminate the existing formula, which takes the median fee of the 56 fee schedules and reduces it by 26 percent to set the NLA, would require new legislation. Thus, a single national fee schedule or any of the alternatives discussed previously would require congressional action. Additional legislation would be required to extend the current competitive bidding demonstration authority and to permit the use of demonstrations for the purposes of developing data with which to set relative values.

Administrative Steps. Under any of the payment options raised earlier in this chapter, administrative changes would be necessary. The committee's goal would be to take advantage of this opportunity to simplify, streamline, and open the administrative procedures whenever possible. Some methods, such as market-based alternatives, would require a very different approach from that required by use of the NLA. The extent of the administrative changes under any approach would depend on how elaborate the procedures were for setting the initial payments and later sets of fees or relative values. A system that began with the NLA would create the opportunity to simplify some administrative procedures by eliminating certain functions related to the 56 carrier fee schedules. Alternatives for refining relative values, for instance, could require policy decisions about research contracts and surveys, how to refine market-based demonstrations, how to structure stakeholders' meetings, and how to solicit public comments. Additional administrative procedures could be required for updating the fee schedule under some alternatives. Incorporating new technologies under certain options could mean reduced administrative activity by the carriers and more work done centrally by HCFA, resulting in greater efficiency.

A change of payment methodology could provide an opportunity for HCFA to address related administrative issues needing attention, such as the clarification of instructions to carriers concerning claims denials, that are not necessarily related to the particular alternative selected. At a time of significant policy changes, it would be particularly important to have all of the stakeholders understand the proposed changes and participate in their refinement, to the extent possible.

Paperwork. Under the fee-for-service alternatives considered in this chapter, there is no reason to expect that the claim form and accompanying data currently required of physicians and laboratories to bill for laboratory services would be changed substantially. New paperwork burdens could result from the studies suggested for planning a new system and monitoring its impact. The extent of the burden would depend on the type of data collection required, study design, survey sample size, and other methodological requirements. As discussed earlier in this chapter, a survey of laboratories to determine the costs per test could be quite complex and demanding of the respondents. A competitive bidding or negotiation demonstration would be relatively less intrusive, but demanding of the laboratories as they calculated their risks and bids. Other research, evaluation, and administrative requirements could create paperwork burdens and costs associated with conducting a demonstration. The paperwork burden of the consensus approach would depend, in part, on the extent of the information incorporated into the process and the method chosen to identify participants in the consensus process.

Financial Costs of Introduction and Use. The initial financial costs of the NLA approach would be minimal because no new data collection would be necessary for calculating the basic fee schedule. Software changes would likely be relatively minor since this would be more a matter of dropping the 56 local fee schedules than of creating totally new systems. The MFN option could require extensive software changes to prepare carriers to pay the laboratories based on their individual charges. The cost of a competitive bidding demonstration would depend on the number of geographic locations and laboratories included. Determinations of what data to use for payment updates and any geographic adjustments, how they should be calculated, and to what costs they should be applied, could draw heavily on existing information. HCFA has had extensive experience in creating such updates and adjustments for other types of providers. The costs of implementing adjustments would depend on how much precision was needed and how much original data collection and modeling would be necessary.

Significant expenses could be incurred for initial calculations of the costs or resource base for alternatives using relative values. There would be costs for calculating certain types of adjustments as well. Depending on how initial relative values are calculated, sufficient data could be produced by the process to contribute to the determination of whether some adjustments should be made. The cost of acquiring the necessary data depends largely on several key design decisions, such as the data collection approach (which affects both data costs and validity) and the type of measure (mean, median, or efficient model) upon which relative values will be based. Ultimately, the costs of developing an RVS would depend on the process chosen for establishing relative values and the amounts and type of data it requires.

CONCLUSION

The choice of a payment alternative does not have to be "either/or"; it could include various options. Incurring the major start-up costs and longer-term redistributive costs of some of the more complex alternatives is presumably reasonable if concerns about inefficiencies, inequities, or access problems with the current system merit the implementation costs and potential disruption associated with them. In the absence of evidence of such problems, it is likely that the industry has accommodated whatever payment distortions there are relative to costs under current policy. In this case, the less expensive, more pragmatic approach of a national fee schedule based on the NLAs may be justifiable as a first step toward a more coherent Medicare laboratory payment policy with minimal short-run implications for the industry or beneficiaries. However, the NLAs could present difficulties if used indefinitely since it is unclear how these fees relate to costs in aggregate or to costs of specific tests. A resource-based fee schedule, set at a reasonable level, would eliminate incentives for providers to limit access to

Medicare beneficiaries. Once the NLA fee schedule is in place, it could be gradually improved so that the fees more closely reflected the relative resource use of each test. This refinement could occur through a consensus process informed by data gathered through the types of approaches described earlier.

There would inevitably be costs related to any policy reform and changes needed in the administration of the program. There would also be costs and potential access problems associated with making no changes, and maintaining the status quo indefinitely into the future. Given current concerns about distortions in payments and constraints on efficiently updating the system, as well as demands on the current payment methodology that will result from new laboratory technologies under development, it is important that HCFA and Congress consider the committee's recommendations in the following chapter. Changes cannot be effected well if done hastily in a crisis situation, so it would be advantageous to begin planning, collecting the needed data, and analyzing them so that a properly designed payment methodology can be developed.

REFERENCES

Axt-Adam, P., J. C. van der Wouden, and E. van der Does. 1993. Influencing behavior of physicians ordering laboratory tests: A literature study. *Med Care* 31, No. 9:784–794.

Brook, R. H., J.E. Ware, Jr., W. H. Rogers, et. al. 1984. *The Effect of Coinsurance on the Health of Adults: Results from the RAND Health Insurance Experiment.* R-3055-HHS. Santa Monica, CA: RAND.

Committee on Ways and Means, U. S. House of Representatives. 1998. *1998 Green Book: Overview of Entitlement Programs.* Washington, DC: Government Printing Office.

Congressional Budget Office (CBO). 2000. Budget Options. Web page, accessed April 2000. Available at http://www.cbo.gov/.

DeParle, N. M., and R. A. Berenson. 2000. The need for demonstrations to test new ideas. *Health Affairs* 19, No. 5:57-59.

Hindmarsh, J. T., and A. W. Lyon. 1996. Strategies to promote rational clinical chemistry test utilization [see comments]. *Clin Biochem* 29, No. 4:291–299.Comment in *Clin Biochem* 1997; 30, No. 4:361, 363.

Hoerger, T. J., and T. M. Waters. 1993. Competitive bidding for Medicare services. *Med Care* 31, No. 10:879–897.

Hoerger, T. J., J. L. Eggleston, E. Basker, and R. C. Lindrooth. 1997. *Background Report on the Clinical Laboratory Industry, Final Report.* Research Triangle Park, NC: Research Triangle Institute.

McAfee, R. P., and J. McMillan. 1987. Auctions and bidding. *Journal of Economic Literature* 25, No. 2:699-738.

Mennemeyer, S. 1989. Competitive bidding for Medicare outpatient laboratory tests. *Advances in Health Economics and Health Services Research* 10:313–333.

Mennemeyer, S. T., J. B. Christianson, R. Englbrecht-Wiggins, and P. Chemawat. 1986. *Competitive Bidding for Durable Medical Equipment and Clinical Laboratory Services: A Review of Related Literature.* Prepared under contract No. HCFA 500-85-0052. Cambridge, MA: ABT Associates, Inc.

Oliver, T. 1993. Analysis, advice, and congressional leadership: The Physician Payment Review Commission and the politics of Medicare. *Journal of Health Politics, Policy and Law* 18, No. 1:114–174.

Physician Payment Review Commission (PPRC). 1989. *Annual Report to Congress, 1989*. Washington, D.C.: PPRC.

PPRC. 1995. *Annual Report to Congress 1995*. Washington, D.C.: PPRC.

The President's FY 2001 Budget Proposal. Web page, accessed April 2000. Available at http://whitehouse.gov/WH/New/00Budget.

Raslavicus, PA. January 20, 2000. Statement to the IOM Committee on Medicare Payment Methodology for Clinical Laboratory Services. Washington, DC.

Root, C. January 20, 2000. Testimony before the IOM Committee on Medicare Payment Methodology for Clinical Laboratory Services. Washington, DC.

Sing, M., R. Brown, and S. C. Hill. 1998. The consequences of paying Medicare managed care plans their costs. *Inquiry* 35, No. 2:210–222.

Smith, D. G. 1992. *Paying for Medicare: The Politics of Reform*. New York: de Gruyter.

Solanki, G., and H. H. Schauffler. 1999. Cost-sharing and the utilization of clinical preventive services. *Am J Prev Med* 17, No. 2:127–133.

Solanki, G., H. H. Schauffler, and L. S. Miller. 2000. The direct and indirect effects of cost-sharing on the use of preventive services. *Health Serv Res* 34, No. 6:1331–1350.

van Walraven, C., and C. D. Naylor. 1998. Do we know what inappropriate laboratory utilization is? A systematic review of laboratory clinical audits [see comments]. *JAMA* 280, No. 6:550–558.Comment in *JAMA* 1998 ;280, No. 6:565-566.

7

Recommendations

INTRODUCTION

After analyzing the current payment method and alternative policies, the committee reached consensus on 12 recommendations for improving the Medicare system for outpatient clinical laboratory services (see Box 7.1 for a summary of the recommendations). The committee's choices were guided by its previously stated goals for an optimal payment system. The committee considered administrative, legislative, and financial steps necessary to implement alternative payment methods. The committee's recommendations provide broad, general policy guidance. The details regarding how recommendations are implemented could have a significant impact on ultimate system costs.

The first six recommendations are interrelated and cascade from the first recommendation, which broadly defines the preferred payment system and flows into more detailed recommendations concerning specific elements of the system and its implementation. The first six recommendations focus specifically on payment methodology. They address issues such as how to establish the relative value of one test versus another and how to determine the relative resource use of different tests. They do not, however, reflect a conclusion about whether current Medicare aggregate payments or the payment for a particular test is too high or too low.

The final six recommendations focus on problems in the current system. These recommendations can be implemented independently or concurrently with the first six. They consider such issues as the structure of the claims-processing contractors and how to improve payment-related administrative procedures.

BOX 7.1 Recommendations

Because changes in the current Medicare payment formula could require new legislation, implementation of many of the committee's recommendations will entail congressional action. The committee recommends that the Health Care Financing Administration (HCFA), the administration, and the Congress work together to develop the necessary enabling authority and funding.

Recommendation 1: Medicare payments for outpatient clinical laboratory services should be based on a single, rational, national fee schedule.

Recommendation 2: On an interim basis, relative payments for Medicare outpatient clinical laboratory services should be based on the current National Limitation Amounts (NLAs).

Recommendation 3: A data-driven consensus process for refining the new Medicare national fee schedule for outpatient clinical laboratory services should be developed. HCFA should explore alternative methods for gathering data to be used in the process.

Recommendation 4: Medicare national fees for outpatient clinical laboratory services should be adjusted for geographic location. HCFA should also evaluate the need to adjust for certain other circumstances, particularly those likely to affect beneficiary access, and make recommendations to the Congress.

Recommendation 5: Processes should be put in place to refine and periodically update the fee schedule for Medicare outpatient clinical laboratory services.

Recommendation 6: To incorporate new tests into the Medicare laboratory fee schedule, there should be an open, timely, and accessible process that is subject to challenge. The process and fees produced should not impede clinical decision making that is essential to providing appropriate care.

Recommendation 7: HCFA should review alternatives to the current system for coding outpatient clinical laboratory services for claims processing. More accurate, open, and timely coding processes for new technologies as well as tests and services should be sought.

Recommendation 8: The current policy of not requiring beneficiary cost sharing for Medicare outpatient clinical laboratory services should continue. Cost sharing is unlikely to significantly reduce overuse or increase the detection of fraud and abuse; it could create barriers to access for the most vulnerable Medicare beneficiaries; and it would be financially and administratively burdensome for laboratories, patients, and the Medicare program depending on its design.

Recommendation 9: HCFA should discontinue use of International Classification of Diseases, Ninth Revision (ICD-9) diagnosis codes as the basis for determining the medical necessity of clinical laboratory tests. HCFA should assess the need for any approach to evaluating the medical necessity of individual laboratory tests prior to payment of a claim. In addition, HCFA should evaluate alternative approaches for identifying and reducing unnecessary or inappropriate laboratory testing.

Continued

BOX 7.1 *Continued*

Recommendation 10: In its policy formulation processes, HCFA should provide opportunities for stakeholder input and develop better communication with contractors and other stakeholders when policies are being developed and once they are adopted.

Recommendation 11: HCFA should move promptly to consolidate the number of contractors processing all Medicare outpatient clinical laboratory claims, including claims from physician office laboratories (POLs) and hospital-based laboratories. The design of this consolidation should ensure that claims processing by regional laboratory carriers will not require major new billing procedures for POLs or hospital-based laboratories. Efforts should be made to strengthen local provider services and relations between carriers and laboratories.

Recommendation 12: HCFA should collect the data needed to effectively manage the performance of the Medicare outpatient clinical laboratory payment system.

RECOMMENDATION 1: Medicare payments for outpatient clinical laboratory services should be based on a single, rational, national fee schedule.

The committee concluded that there is already, in effect, a national fee schedule, since a very significant share of services are actually paid at the national cap (Appendix B). Continuing to maintain 56 regional fee schedules that pay essentially national fees makes payment policy unclear to stakeholders and perpetuates an unnecessary burden of administering the system. Current Medicare payment policies for ambulatory laboratory services are unnecessarily complicated. Although the committee found no sound evidence that these policies currently pose a threat to beneficiary access,[1] they have become increasingly cumbersome both to the clinical laboratories that provide services to Medicare beneficiaries and to the Health Care Financing Administration (HCFA) and its contractors.

A national fee schedule allows the establishment of a single set of payments for all outpatient clinical laboratory services, adjustments for differences in local labor costs and prices for goods and services the laboratory purchases, and if appropriate, other relevant factors. Ideally, a payment for a test or service should reflect some notion of the relative value of resources required to produce it. That is, if Test A for one condition generally costs laboratories twice as much to produce as does Test B for another condition, the payment for Test A should be twice as much as that for Test B. This concept of resource-based relative values is important for a national fee schedule, since Medicare's payments should not create financial incentives to provide certain services or withhold others. The current

[1]See discussion in Chapter 5.

system of capped regional payments is not based on relative resource requirements, which could distort the price signals to providers, both across geographic areas and from test to test within each jurisdiction. The current system could ultimately compromise the appropriateness of care available to beneficiaries.

The long-term goal for the single national outpatient clinical laboratory fee schedule is to establish payment amounts that accurately reflect the relative costs of services, minimizing the financial incentives to overuse or underuse services. Once a single national fee schedule is established, there ought to be regional adjustments to it. This is generally necessary in national payment systems because there are regional differences in input prices such as labor and supplies that could affect the cost of delivering laboratory services.

The committee considers this long-term goal of a resource-based national fee schedule important both for promoting clinically appropriate use of laboratory services and for ensuring that beneficiaries can have access to services. The key building blocks of such a fee schedule include (1) a relative value scale (RVS); (2) a dollar conversion factor that translates these relative values into payment amounts; (3) any adjustments for laboratory, beneficiary, or other characteristics such as geographic location; and (4) periodic updates.

The small amount of laboratory payments as a share of Medicare payments to all providers and suppliers, 1.6 percent, has made the committee question the wisdom of undergoing an expensive, extended study before moving toward a new national schedule. For the same reason, and because the current system does seem to provide the access beneficiaries need, the committee rejected the option of moving to any payment system that is radically different from the current fee schedule and could entail a complex, time-consuming transition and major dislocations. As a result, the committee makes specific additional recommendations about how to move quickly to a national fee schedule and then develop a process for refining and improving it that balances potential improvements against additional development costs.

RECOMMENDATION 2: On an interim basis, relative payments for Medicare outpatient clinical laboratory services should be based on the current National Limitation Amounts (NLAs).

The NLAs are an appropriate starting point for creating a national fee schedule, but HCFA should move quickly to refine them. There is no obvious relationship between the NLAs and relative costs; however, the committee concluded that there are several reasons to use NLAs as a first step toward developing a national, rational fee schedule. First, moving to a national fee schedule based on the NLAs simply formalizes what has already become de facto Medicare outpatient laboratory payments. Second, using the NLAs as a starting point for a new national fee schedule should minimize dislocations for laboratories, beneficiaries, and contractors. The NLAs are already essentially a national fee schedule, so official adoption of NLAs in this capacity should cause minimal disruptions for stakeholders. This is important to the committee primarily because of the apparent lack of beneficiary access problems under the current payment system. Finally, the very limited evidence available suggests that current Medicare payment rates are generally within the range of those of other payers, in terms of both relative values and dollar amounts (Appendix C). Regardless of whether this occurs because other payers follow Medicare's lead in pricing or for some other reason, it suggests that Medicare's rates have some degree of face validity within the industry. It appears that Medicare payments generally are within the range of market prices at which laboratories are willing to sell their services.

The committee had no basis, beyond the discussions in Chapter 5 and above, to determine whether Medicare should increase, decrease, or maintain the current level of aggregate spending on outpatient clinical laboratory services. In any case, it makes sense to move to a single, national fee schedule, starting with the NLAs.

Under current law, there will be no Medicare outpatient clinical laboratory fee increase or decrease through 2002. If the Congress and HCFA were to maintain this requirement while implementing the new fee schedule (i.e., projected aggregate outpatient clinical laboratory spending under Medicare remains the same), then it is an inescapable conclusion that current NLA levels would have to be slightly reduced across the board to permit the carrier fees currently below the NLAs to rise.

A preliminary analysis conducted for the committee suggests that a reduction of the NLAs as little as 1 or 2 percentage points may be sufficient to maintain the current level of aggregate spending (Appendix B). More detailed, accurate analyses of this issue would have to be conducted before the exact amount of the change could be determined. If those studies suggest that a markedly larger reduction in the NLAs would be needed if the Congress were to call for maintaining budget neutrality, the committee suggests that the new fee schedule be phased in over two or more years, to minimize disruptions experienced by beneficiaries and clinical laboratories.

RECOMMENDATION 3: A data-driven consensus process for refining the new Medicare national fee schedule for outpatient clinical laboratory services should be developed. HCFA should explore alternative methods for gathering data to be used in the process.

The committee believes that a data-driven consensus approach is most likely to be a practical and successful approach to refining the fee schedule. HCFA should examine the costs, potential value, strengths, and weaknesses of other approaches and alternative methods for gathering data on costs and developing relative values before refining or replacing the NLA-based fee schedule.

Several interdisciplinary groups could, through an interactive process, either review and refine the NLA-based fee schedule or develop a completely new set of relative values. The process could be used for changing selected fees that are noticeably out of line with respect to resource use or could focus attention on those tests that contribute most to Medicare spending. Alternatively, the process could be used for a comprehensive analysis of every test or groups of similar tests. Such an analytical approach was used to refine physician work values and establish practice expense values for the physician fee schedule. This approach would be built around the participation of laboratorians, as well as other stakeholders. Such a process could use data from many sources in a systematic and rigorous way.

A consensus approach could lend legitimacy and credibility to the newly developed values if it is designed in a manner acceptable to stakeholders. Unless care is taken in its design, however, it is vulnerable to criticisms about the process for identifying participants, the method for combining information from different sources, and the possible impropriety of using subjective, qualitative methods to measure what some think should be readily quantifiable. If the focus of the refinement effort is the actual fees rather than their relative values, this method would have to include budget constraints or it could be inflationary. In fact, the parameters for setting the initial conversion factor, which would define the level of payment for the relative value scale, would likely be specified by the Congress.

The committee considered a number of approaches for establishing resource-based relative payment rates.[2] Each approach has some advantages and disadvantages; specific risks, potential disruptions, and different consequences depending on how it is designed. These approaches are not mutually exclusive and could be combined in various ways to facilitate the refinement of the NLAs or the creation of a new national fee schedule. Elements of different basic approaches could be combined to maximize the advantages and minimize the disadvantages, including costs. For example, some limited, detailed cost studies could provide a basis for rigorous analysis by consensus groups. Four approaches merit further consideration:

- **Micro-costing studies:** HCFA would collect objective cost data related to specific services from laboratories, manufacturers, and other appropriate sources. The research could entail detailed cost-accounting studies to identify costs associated with each laboratory service, or it could consist of smaller studies targeted at selected tests. The costs would include that of technicians, pathologists, clinical experts and other labor, equipment, and supplies, transportation, and administrative functions, such as regulatory compliance associated with the production of laboratory tests. Likewise, this approach could range from the use of a random, stratified sample of all laboratories to the use of smaller samples of average or efficient laboratories from which to gather cost data. In any case, high-quality data would require careful study design, clearly defined methods for collecting consistent cost data, and mandatory participation. A well-done study of this type could result in accurate, detailed cost data, but it would be relatively expensive.

---

[2]See Chapter 6.

• **Competitive bidding demonstration:** A competitive bidding demonstration could provide a basis for national relative values. It should be designed primarily to elicit accurate information about market pricing rather than to purchase services. Submitted bids should reveal the cost of production and, therefore, could be used as the basis for establishing relative values. However, the use of bids made under the assumption that the laboratory would receive increased volume from Medicare could be misleading if they were taken as indicative of resource-based prices when setting fees that would apply to all laboratories. HCFA is developing experience with competitive bidding in other service areas and is planning a regional demonstration for outpatient clinical laboratory fees. If this takes place, the data derived from it would be useful to the consensus process. Data obtained from regional demonstrations would have to be adjusted for national application since the committee does not support bidding on a national level.

• **Negotiated fee demonstration:** A demonstration in selected areas, based on a private sector model of negotiation, could be used by carriers and area laboratories to agree on a fee schedule. Like competitive bidding, this approach also provides a basis for developing relative values. Again, data would be regional rather than national. Some Medicare carriers have institutional experience with negotiating for their private plans, but it is unclear how much of this expertise could be shared with their Medicare staff. Similarly, some laboratories have experience negotiating with payers, but it is unclear how common this is, particularly among smaller laboratories.

• **Charges:** The charges employed by laboratories on each Medicare claim could contribute to the development of relative values. This option is simple since it is based on available data. It is not clear, however, how closely current charges reflect costs since the committee has found no published studies of laboratory costs and charges. If an alternative approach were used to collect cost data or determine relative resource use, it would be helpful to compare these data to charges from claims, because, if charges were shown to be consistently related, claims could prove an easy and inexpensive data source for future revisions.

The committee recommends that HCFA examine the costs, potential value, strengths, and weaknesses of these approaches and other methods for developing resource-based relative values before refining or replacing the NLA-based fee schedule. Researchers, industry leaders, policy experts, and others should be included in the agency's efforts to compare these alternatives and assess their appropriateness for contributing useful data that could be used in the development of relative values for clinical laboratory services.

RECOMMENDATION 4: Medicare national fees for outpatient clinical laboratory services should be adjusted for geographic location. HCFA should also evaluate the need to adjust for certain other circumstances, particularly those likely to affect beneficiary access, and make recommendations to the Congress.

Some costs, primarily labor and specimen transportation costs, may vary widely across the nation and between urban and rural areas. Current differences in the 56 carrier fee schedules may reflect, at least to some degree, such variation, although they are not for the most part passed along through Medicare payments because of the widespread use of NLAs.[3] It would be appropriate to have some systematic geographic adjuster for these costs. HCFA has had extensive experience with this issue since geographic adjusters have been incorporated into virtually all of Medicare's prospective payment systems, including its capitation payments.

Generally, the committee does not support adjustments based on broad categories of laboratories, such as physician office, hospital-based, or independent laboratories, unless there is evidence of significant cost differences and problems affecting beneficiary access. The committee has discussed a number of provider, test, and beneficiary characteristics that may be associated with cost differences and should be reflected in Medicare payments. It is most concerned with situations in which lack of adjustment to national fees is likely to affect beneficiaries' ability to obtain needed services.

The committee recommends that HCFA also study cost differences associated with the following:

- **Qualified laboratories in sole community hospitals:**[4] These providers currently receive slightly higher Medicare outpatient laboratory payments. HCFA should study the implications for sole community hospitals of a new national fee schedule. It should determine whether these hospital-based laboratories generally are likely to benefit from a national fee schedule or whether some additional percentage payment during transition or over a longer term is needed to maintain access for the beneficiaries traditionally served by these providers.
- **STAT tests:** The committee recognizes that tests that must be conducted immediately for urgent or emergency care may present additional costs that may have to be recognized by Medicare payments. The committee was unable to find any data to document whether these tests are, in fact, markedly more costly, so it recommends that HCFA study this issue further. If there is a need to recognize STAT tests in Medicare payments, care should be taken with the way in which STAT circumstances are defined and monitored in order to minimize inappropriate use of the STAT designation.

---

[3]Fees that are below the NLAs are an artifact of charge data from the early 1980s and may, in fact, be lower because costs were lower in those regions. Regions that have unusually high costs are not accommodated in the current payment system because the NLAs put an upper limit on the payment rate.

[4]A sole community hospital is located 25–35 miles from similar hospitals, serves at least 75 percent of the local residents needing such inpatient care, and meets the detailed criteria contained in 42 C.F.R. 412.92. A qualified laboratory in a sole community hospital is one that provides some clinical diagnostic tests 24 hours a day, seven days a week, in order to serve the hospital's emergency room, which is available around the clock.

RECOMMENDATION 5: Processes should be put in place to refine and periodically update the fee schedule for Medicare outpatient clinical laboratory services.

To remain viable, the national fee schedule must respond to economic and scientific changes that affect the cost of providing services. A new national fee schedule for laboratory services would require periodic review and refinement, regardless of the method used initially to establish resource-based relative values. Explicit processes that include opportunities for public input, review, and challenge should be established. Procedures may vary for different elements or building blocks of the fee schedule. For example, an annual process should be established for updating the conversion factor so that it is appropriate relative to inflation, changes in the size and composition of the beneficiary population, changes in laboratory technology, or other appropriate factors. Similarly, an approach should also be articulated for reviewing and updating any adjustments, such as geographic differences in input prices, on a regular basis. Finally, a clear process should be developed for the review of relative values every few years. This periodic review would provide an opportunity to recalibrate the fee schedule to reflect important changes in laboratory operations and technology and to refine values of new technologies. The processes for incorporating new test methodologies and technologies are discussed in Recommendation 6.

• **Update factor:** The update or conversion factor could be applied across the board to the current NLAs or to a fee schedule that is based on relative values. Initially, a conversion factor would have to be established to translate the laboratory relative values into dollar amounts. After the first year, the conversion factor should be updated annually.

The process for updating the fee schedule should identify the responsible parties, the schedule for acquiring and analyzing data, and the factors that should be considered in developing the updated amount. Because the update factor will affect federal spending, it is likely to be established through the annual budget process. Although HCFA would ultimately be responsible for implementing updated rates, it might be appropriate to require the Medicare Payment Advisory Commission (MedPAC) or another suitable government agency to make recommendations to the Congress about the update factor. Since laboratory service volume growth is already included in the sustainable growth rate (SGR) process used to calculate updates to physician payment rates, reflecting the role physicians play in ordering the tests performed by laboratories, it should not play a role in updating laboratory payments.[5]

• **Payment adjustments:** Review and revision of geographic and other payment adjustments should include analyses of their effect on beneficiary access to laboratory services. To the extent that adjusters for local price variation or STAT services may be important for maintaining access to services, under-

---

[5]See Chapter 5.

standing their effectiveness requires some information about access. For any adjusters ultimately included, a process for reviewing and revising them as necessary should be developed.

• **Relative values:** Periodic review of the relative values, however they were originally established, is essential for maintaining the integrity of the recommended payment approach. The relative costs of existing services change over time as new methods and equipment become available and other workplace and scientific innovations affect the way in which services are performed. As a result, periodic review of all services, not just new ones, is necessary to correct values where such changes have occurred. The review process for relative values should be defined to make explicit potential trade-offs within constrained resources. In fact, the changes in relative values for particular tests should be made under an assumption of budget neutrality since the update factor would be applied annually to all tests equally.

These various processes are essential to the continued appropriateness of the Medicare laboratory payment system over time. Without them, the key elements of the payment methodology may become inconsistent with the original design intent.

RECOMMENDATION 6: To incorporate new tests into the Medicare laboratory fee schedule, there should be an open, timely, and accessible process that is subject to challenge. The process and fees produced should not impede clinical decision making that is essential to providing appropriate care.

The committee has concluded that a consistent, public process for developing interim values for new laboratory services is essential for an effective payment system. Such a process could improve current methods used to establish payment rates for new services and address many of the concerns stakeholders have about current policy. Data to support this process could be gathered from various sources including the HCFA contractors, private payers, laboratories, and manufacturers.

Central to this process, HCFA should create a committee of laboratorians, pathologists, other physicians and scientific experts, health services policymakers, and economists to advise on the setting of interim relative values or national fees for new technologies. There should be an open process for determining which technologies are truly innovative and sufficiently different from existing ones to merit a detailed cost analysis and new fee, and which new tests and methods are incremental improvements and could be paid at the same rate as an existing test. The manufacturer and others should be allowed to present data to the committee showing quantifiable improvements in treatment outcomes and other advantages of the new test that might justify a higher payment rate than that of existing, similar tests. After establishing interim values or fees for new services, Medicare should allow a certain time for diffusion of the new technology and stabilization of costs. Before the end of the interim period, the interim fees for these new services should be reviewed and revised as necessary. Once they are "official," these services would be included in the normal periodic review process of relative values for the full fee schedule.

Beyond this, policies should be developed that allow for more timely assignment of codes in the HCFA Common Procedural Coding System (HCPCS). The use of local, temporary, price-appropriate codes set by carriers during the period before a national interim fee could possibly facilitate the introduction of new tests. HCFA should establish clear guidance for its carriers on how to establish payments prior to setting interim prices nationally. The process for incorporating new technology should include public input.

RECOMMENDATION 7: HCFA should review alternatives to the current system for coding outpatient clinical laboratory services for claims processing. More accurate, open, and timely coding processes for new technologies as well as tests and services should be sought.

The committee heard testimony from several sources that the Current Procedural Terminology (CPT) coding process[6] often adds to the time required to incorporate new technologies into the Medicare laboratory payment system. There are also problems with the inadequate specificity of the codes. Coding, the Medicare coverage process, and payment determinations are closely intertwined; tend to lack transparency; and can add considerably to the time required to incorporate a new test, new equipment, or a new testing methodology. The committee is concerned that this problem will be exacerbated in the future, as new technologies for laboratory tests grow at an increasing rate and as the "useful life" of a new technology is shortened by the rapid introduction of newer and improved technologies. HCFA should examine how to reduce coding delays within the current system and examine alternative coding systems distinct from CPT.

RECOMMENDATION 8: The current policy of not requiring beneficiary cost sharing for Medicare outpatient clinical laboratory services should continue. Cost sharing is unlikely to significantly reduce overuse or increase the detection of fraud and abuse; it could create barriers to access for the most vulnerable Medicare beneficiaries; and it would be financially and administratively burdensome for laboratories, patients, and the Medicare program depending on its design.

Originally there was a copayment for Medicare laboratory services, as there was for most other Medicare services. It was eliminated in 1984, with the under-

---

[6]The physicians' coding system, called the Current Procedural Terminology, Fourth Edition (CPT-4), is maintained by the American Medical Association.

standing that the fees established would represent payment in full. The laboratory industry accepted that fees would be somewhat reduced in exchange for not having the administrative costs of billing the beneficiary for generally small copayments.

The committee recognizes the importance of deductibles and copayments in the Medicare program as tools for reducing program expenditures and encouraging the selection of necessary and cost-effective services. Conceptually, cost sharing is expected to reduce overuse of health services by making patients more aware of service costs. For laboratory services, however, the patient does not initiate this use, usually has no contact with the laboratory, often has supplemental insurance that mutes the cost impact, and is unlikely to challenge the physician's order. The medical literature is replete with examples of overuse of laboratory tests in the inpatient hospital setting (Axt-Adam et al., 1993; Hindmarsh and Lyon, 1996; van Walraven and Naylor, 1998). Similar studies on outpatient testing were not found. However, because laboratory tests are requested by a physician (or other health care provider) to aid with the diagnosis or monitoring of a beneficiary's medical condition, the volume of laboratory tests appears to be more sensitive to the number of physician–patient contacts than to the number of tests used per patient contact (Danzon et al., 1984). This is because the physician orders laboratory tests.

There is little empirical evidence about the effect of cost sharing in cases where demand is not initiated by the patient, and theory suggests that its effect on demand would be quite modest. In addition, nearly 90 percent of Medicare beneficiaries have some form of supplemental insurance that covers costs not covered by Medicare. As a result, beneficiaries do not actually pay their cost-sharing requirements directly, so they may not become more price sensitive when a new cost is instituted. The modest savings expected to accrue from behavioral changes from the copayment provision in the administration's FY 2001 budget suggest that HCFA actuaries also assume little effect on service use.

The committee is concerned not only that cost sharing will not help reduce any overuse of services, but also that it could create barriers to appropriate use for some beneficiaries. Previous studies suggest that cost sharing may decrease access to appropriate services and disproportionately burden the poor and chronically ill (Lurie et al., 1989; Shapiro et al., 1986; Solanki and Schauffler, 1999; Solanki et al., 2000; Stuart and Zacker, 1999). It is difficult to know how these findings generalize to the Medicare beneficiary population; nonetheless, the committee is concerned that the 10 percent without supplemental insurance could be in a financially vulnerable situation that might lead them to forgo needed tests.

An additional concern is that cost sharing is unlikely to lead to significant reductions in fraud and abuse. It seems unlikely that beneficiaries will become an important check on the system, since they typically are unaware of the exact type of test ordered or of the laboratory to which their specimen was sent. As a result, they may not be in a position to interpret their Explanation of Medicare Benefits with enough understanding to detect fraud. Historically, inside "whistle-blowers" have been the main sources for detecting fraud and abuse in laboratory services, not Medicare contractors and beneficiaries.

The committee's practical concern has to do with administering a set of deductibles or copayments. Given the relatively low per-service payment amount for common laboratory procedures, a 20 percent copayment would typically be less than about $2.30. In many cases, the cost to the laboratory of billing and collecting the copayment and the associated bad debt would exceed the expected payment amount, particularly since the laboratory otherwise has no direct contact with the beneficiary. Although it may be a reasonable business decision to forgo the copayment in many cases, laboratories would risk charges of billing fraud if they failed to make an effort to collect these payments.[7]

RECOMMENDATION 9: HCFA should discontinue use of International Classification of Diseases, Ninth Revision (ICD-9) diagnosis codes as the basis for determining the medical necessity of clinical laboratory tests. HCFA should assess the need for any approach to evaluating the medical necessity of individual laboratory tests prior to payment of a claim. In addition, HCFA should evaluate alternative approaches for identifying and reducing unnecessary or inappropriate laboratory testing.

Determinations of medical necessity based on diagnosis codes were instituted to improve the appropriateness of testing and, in part, to discourage fraud and abuse related to physician self-referral. Since implementation of the Stark legislation, there has been less financial incentive for physicians to order unnecessary tests.[8] In addition, experience has shown that the use of ICD-9 codes is not a sound basis for making judgments regarding the medical necessity of particular laboratory tests in specific patients.[9] One of the fundamental problems with the approach that the contractors currently use to make a determination of the medical necessity of a particular laboratory test for a particular beneficiary at a particular time is that, in many circumstances, it is likely to give the wrong answer. Moreover, the current system is easily gamed, is administratively burdensome, and does not place sufficient responsibility on the physician.

HCFA has developed a complex system of guidelines, some local and some national, including policies for 23 common tests, that advise physicians on what diagnosis codes constitute appropriate use of particular tests. The national policies for these 23 tests, recently developed under a negotiated rulemaking process (Neg Reg), potentially are a considerable improvement over the many conflict-

---

[7]See Chapter 6 for further discussion.

[8]The Ethics in Patient Referral Act, enacted in 1989, is named after the legislation's sponsor, Representative F. Pete Stark, and restricts physicians from referring their patients to laboratories in which they or their family members have a financial interest.

[9]The ICD-9 code is a five-digit number indicating the diagnosis or symptoms of a patient.

ing local medical review policies that were in existence. The Neg Reg initiative, however, did not consider the underlying question of whether ICD-9 codes are a sound basis for determining medical necessity. The current system, although commendable in its intentions, is not effective in accomplishing its purpose. It creates a substantial administrative burden on laboratories and physicians, and the need for Medicare and its contractors to develop medical review policies to guide payment determinations.

HCFA currently can document neither the extent nor the nature of denied claims and medically unnecessary testing from its claims processing data. HCFA should monitor laboratory test trends to identify increases in unnecessary tests if they occur. As a prudent buyer, HCFA should examine a number of other approaches for promoting clinically appropriate use of laboratory tests including the following:

- inclusion of outpatient clinical laboratory tests in the peer review organizations' (PROs') next scope of work;
- focused medical reviews of both prepayment and post payment, by contractors or PROs;
- development of approaches for identifying the inappropriate use of laboratory tests supported by the Agency for Healthcare Research and Quality (AHRQ);
- development of methods for holding physicians financially accountable for claims determined to be medically unnecessary; and
- creation of methods to detect and address fraud and abuse developed in conjunction with with the Office of the Inspector General (OIG).

The committee recognizes that this recommendation will make it difficult to know when a patient Advanced Beneficiary Notice (ABN) is necessary. HCFA will have to consider alternative ways of determining whether the patient should be responsible for the bill.

RECOMMENDATION 10: In its policy formulation processes, HCFA should provide opportunities for stakeholder input and develop better communication with contractors and other stakeholders when policies are being developed and once they are adopted.

Many laboratory industry concerns about the Medicare payment system have their origins in the current lack of public input to many current processes and inadequate communication of policy decisions.

Some of the previous recommendations made by the committee address selected aspects of current policymaking that need improvement. For example, the recommendation to develop processes for incorporating new technologies into the fee schedule is due in part to concerns about the current practices of cross-walking and gap-filling values for new tests, both methods currently used for establishing a payment amount for new technology.[10]

There are other areas, however, in which the committee is making no specific recommendation, but where current policies are not clearly explained in easily obtainable written format. For example, clear statements of local medical review policies (LMRPs) of carriers are not always widely available to stakeholders. Recent efforts to move these policies to the Web represent an improvement, but it is sometimes difficult to find policies relevant to a particular service in a particular carrier's service area. Similarly, it is unclear to providers whether and under what conditions laboratories are allowed to bill referring physicians for services provided to Medicare beneficiaries that have been denied Medicare payment.

In the course of its fact-finding activities, the committee uncovered potentially useful information that was not widely known by affected stakeholders. For example, representatives of the laboratory industry and many physicians are unaware of the fact that laboratory service volumes are included in the SGR system used to update physician payments under the Medicare physician fee schedule. If laboratory service volume grows more than expected, then physician payment rates will grow more slowly. The fact that key stakeholders were unaware of the inclusion of laboratory services in this SGR system suggests that the potential incentives of the system have been muted.

These examples suggest the need for HCFA and its contractors to communicate more effectively with stakeholders about both national and local policies. The committee recommends that HCFA develop a method for accomplishing this to ensure that laboratories, referring physicians, and beneficiaries have easier access to information about the laws, policies, and procedures that affect their ability to provide and receive clinical laboratory services and receive payment for them.

RECOMMENDATION 11: HCFA should move promptly to consolidate the number of contractors processing all Medicare outpatient clinical laboratory claims, including claims from physician office laboratories (POLs) and hospital-based laboratories. The design of this consolidation should ensure that claims processing by regional laboratory carriers will not require major new billing procedures for POLs or hospital-based laboratories. Efforts should be made to strengthen local provider services and relations between carriers and laboratories.

The committee believes that standardization of program operations is an important aspect of the goal of administrative simplicity and efficiency. Thus, it supports the 1997 Balanced Budget Act section that mandates consolidation of the processing of clinical laboratory claims into four or five regional carriers and

---

[10]See Chapters 4 and 5.

designation of one of the carriers to serve as the central statistical resource, and it encourages HCFA to implement this. The consolidation should create a more efficient and fair administrative process for Medicare laboratory payments.

The committee found that HCFA's current administrative process of working through 56 carrier regions, with approximately 23 distinct carriers and 30 fiscal intermediaries (FIs), creates inconsistencies in the interpretation of HCFA policy and procedures, duplicates the cost of pricing new tests, and leads to variable interpretations of medical necessity for the same tests. These inconsistencies can cause particular problems for laboratories that perform tests on specimens drawn from beneficiaries in many different states since the laboratories may have to deal with differing policies and procedures for each claim. The large number of carriers and FIs contributes to a reduced ability to detect broad patterns of fraud, waste, and abuse that extend beyond state boundaries. In addition, with the recommended move to a national fee schedule, the rationale for maintaining a carrier role for the development of local gap-fill fees is eliminated. Because the rate of diffusion of new tests and technologies varies by locale, the regional laboratory carriers (RLCs) would carry on the role of deciding coverage and pricing for new technologies until diffusion is sufficient nationally to support HCFA headquarters making national coverage determinations and prices for them.

The committee recognizes that many design questions must be resolved in planning for this consolidation of laboratory claims-processing functions and considers that it would not be worth the substantial expense of consolidation unless all outpatient laboratory claims were processed through RLCs. To avoid inconvenience to POLs and to hospitals billing for their outpatient laboratories, however, it is important to design a mechanism by which they can continue to submit bills to their carriers and FIs, respectively, which could then forward the laboratory portion of the claim to the RLCs. Recognizing that this route for providers of following familiar administrative procedures would likely add time to the payment process, HCFA could also offer POLs and hospital-based laboratories the alternative of submitting laboratory claims directly to the RLCs. Compensating data analysis efforts might also be necessary to permit the examination of all claims associated with an episode of care. Given the scope of this mandated change and the number of design issues yet to be decided, the committee cautions HCFA to monitor change closely and beware of unintended consequences.

RECOMMENDATION 12: HCFA should collect the data needed to effectively manage the performance of the Medicare outpatient clinical laboratory payment system.

HCFA should collect baseline data to inform future policy considerations and additional data to measure the impact of policies, particularly on beneficiary access to care and on the diffusion of new technologies. The committee found no data that indicated directly whether or not current payment policy has resulted in beneficiary access problems. Whenever payment policy is changed, however, policymakers have to monitor for intended and unintended consequences. For example, if Medicare moves to resource-based payments, some segments of the laboratory industry or geographic areas could be more strongly affected than others. Over time, this could change the availability of laboratory services for Medicare beneficiaries. To learn more about these potential access problems and to evaluate the impact of future payment policy changes, the committee recommends that HCFA use existing data sources, such as Clinical Laboratory Improvement Amendments (CLIA) certification, claims data, and the Current Beneficiary Survey, in addition to developing supplemental survey sources to gather direct information concerning harm to patients due to lack of access. Objectives and illustrative examples of baseline and performance measures related to the payment system goals set out by the committee include the following:

- **Beneficiary access**—*Objective:* Determine whether beneficiaries and physicians have adequate access to laboratory services. Possible measures include a sample survey of beneficiaries and physicians to obtain their assessment of any access problems and tracking changes in the number and distribution of laboratories participating in Medicare.
- **Flexibility**—*Objective:* Determine the effectiveness of methods to assign payments for new tests, adjust unreasonable fees, and update payment amounts. Possible measures include a comparison of Medicare and private payments for a broad sample of tests and health plans and tracking the average time needed to adjust unreasonable fees once they have been identified.
- **Transparency**—*Objective:* Determine how well stakeholders understand the processes for setting payment policies and their perceived ability to influence policies. Possible measures include a sample survey of laboratorians, carriers, and physicians to assess their knowledge and perceptions of HCFA's policy processes.
- **Value**—*Objective:* Determine the quality and cost of outpatient laboratory tests purchased by Medicare. Possible measures include monitoring CLIA certification and performance status and claims denial rates, reasons for the denials, and the percentage of claims ultimately paid.
- **Administrative simplicity and efficiency**—*Objective:* Determine how well the key payment processes work within HCFA and in a sample of laboratories, physician practices, and contractors. Possible measures include a comparison of basic processes within contractors to assess their relative efficiency.

CONCLUSION

Congress and HCFA have the opportunity to fix the current payment system for clinical laboratory services, averting the possibility of a crisis in the future. Payments for some individual tests likely do not reflect the cost of providing services, and anticipated advances in laboratory technology will exacerbate the flaws in the current system. Problems with the outdated payment system could threaten beneficiary access to care and the use of enhanced testing methods in the future, although the committee found no evidence of this now. Although radical changes are not called for at this time, implementing the committee's recommendations would likely improve the efficiency of the system and ensure that Medicare beneficiaries continue to have access to high-quality laboratory services.

REFERENCES

Axt-Adam, P., J. C. van der Wouden, and E. van der Does. 1993. Influencing behavior of physicians ordering laboratory tests: A literature study. *Med Care* 31, No. 9:784–794.

Danzon, P. M., W. G. Manning, Jr., and M. S. Marquis. 1984. Factors affecting laboratory test use and prices. *Health Care Financ Rev* 5, No. 4:23–32.

Hindmarsh, J. T., and A. W. Lyon. 1996. Strategies to promote rational clinical chemistry test utilization [see comments]. *Clin Biochem* 29, No. 4:291–299. Comment in *Clin Biochem* 1997; 30, No. 4:361, 363.

Lurie, N., C. J. Kamberg, R. H. Brook, E. B. Keeler, and J. P. Newhouse. 1989. How free care improved vision in the health insurance experiment [published erratum appears in *Am J Public Health* 1989; 79, No. 12:1677]. *Am J Public Health* 79, No. 5:640–642.

Shapiro, M. F., J. E. Ware, Jr., and C. D. Sherbourne. 1986. Effects of cost sharing on seeking care for serious and minor symptoms: Results of a randomized controlled trial. *Ann Intern Med* 104, No. 2:246–251.

Solanki, G., and H. H. Schauffler. 1999. Cost-sharing and the utilization of clinical preventive services. *Am J Prev Med* 17, No. 2:127–133.

Solanki, G., H. H. Schauffler, and L. S. Miller. 2000. The direct and indirect effects of cost-sharing on the use of preventive services. *Health Serv Res* 34, No. 6:1331–1350.

Stuart, B., and C. Zacker. 1999. Who bears the burden of Medicaid drug copayment policies? *Health Aff (Millwood)* 18, No. 2:201–212.

van Walraven, C., and C. D. Naylor. 1998. Do we know what inappropriate laboratory utilization is? A systematic review of laboratory clinical audits [see comments]. *JAMA* 280, no. 6:550–558. Comment in *JAMA* 1998; 280, (6):565–566.

Acronyms and Glossary

ACRONYMS

ABN	Advanced Beneficiary Notice
ACLA	American Clinical Laboratory Association
AHRQ	Agency for Healthcare Research and Quality
AMA	American Medical Association
AST	aspartate transominase
BBA	Balanced Budget Act, 1997
BBRA	Balanced Budget Refinement Act, 1999
CAC	Carrier Advisory Committee
CAGR	compound annual growth rate
CBO	Congressional Budget Office
CDC	Centers for Disease Control and Prevention
CHPS	Center for Health Policy Studies, Columbia, Maryland
CK	creatine kinase
CLIA	Clinical Laboratory Improvement Act, 1967; Clinical Laboratory Improvement Amendments, 1988
CLMA	Clinical Laboratory Management Association
COBRA	Consolidated Omnibus Budget Reconciliation Act, 1985
CPEP	Clinical Practice Expense Panel
CPI	Consumer Price Index
CPK	creatine phosphokinase
CPT	Current Procedural Terminology
CSC	Central Statistical Carrier
CY	calendar year

DEFRA	Deficit Reduction Act, 1984
DHHS	Department of Health and Human Services
DME	durable medical equipment
DNA	deoxyribonucleic acid
DRG	diagnosis-related group
EIA	enzyme immunoassay
EKG	Electrocardiogram
ESRD	end-stage renal disease
FDA	Food and Drug Administration
FI	fiscal intermediary
FMR	focused medical review
FY	fiscal year
GAO	General Accounting Office
GGT	γ-glutamyl transferase
HCFA	Health Care Financing Administration
HCG	human chorionic gonadotropin
HCPCS	HCFA Common Procedural Coding System
HIMA	Health Industry Manufacturers Association, now AdvaMed
HIV	human immunodeficiency virus
HMO	health maintenance organization
HPSA	health professional shortage area
ICD-9-CM	International Classification of Diseases, Ninth Revision, Clinical Modification
Ig	Immunoglobulin
IOM	Institute of Medicine
IT	information technology
LIS	Library Information System
LMRP	local medical review policy
MCAC	Medicare Coverage Advisory Committee
MedPAC	Medicare Payment Advisory Commission
MFN	most favored nation
MIC	minimum inhibitory concentration
Neg Reg	negotiated rulemaking process
NLA	National Limitation Amount
OBRA	Omnibus Budget Reconciliation Act of 1980
OIG	Office of Inspector General, (DHHS)
OMB	Office of Management and Budget
OSHA	Occupational Safety and Health Administration
PCR	polymerase chain reaction
PMA	Pre-Market Approval (FDA)
POCT	point-of-care testing
POL	physician office laboratory
POS	point of service
PMPM	per member per month
PPE	personal protective equipment

PPM	provider performed microscopy
PPO	preferred provider organization
PPRC	Physician Payment Review Commission
PPS	prospective payment system
PRO	peer review organization
PSA	prostate-specific antigen
PT	proficiency testing
QA/QC	quality assurance/quality control
RBC	red blood cell
RBRVS	Resource-based relative value scale
RLC	regional laboratory carrier
RUC	RVS Update Committee
RVS	relative value scale
SGOT	serum glutamic-oxalvacetic transaminase
SGPT	serum glutamic-pyruvic transaminase
SGR	sustainable growth rate
SIC	Standard Industrial Classification
SNF	skilled nursing facility
SSA	Social Security Act, Social Security Administration
TAT	turnaround time
TSH	thyroid-stimulating hormone
UCR	usual, customary, and reasonable
VA	Department of Veterans Affairs
WBC	white blood cell

GLOSSARY

Accession: The process of identifying a specimen and entering a unique specimen identifier into laboratory records.

Accredited laboratory: A laboratory that has voluntarily applied for and been accredited by a private, nonprofit accreditation organization approved by HCFA in accordance with 42 CFR Part 493.

Add-on test: A test ordered on the same sample after the initial tests have been conducted.

Advanced Beneficiary Notice: A written form used to notify a beneficiary, prior to being tested, that Medicare may deny payment if the test is not medically necessary and the beneficiary will be financially responsible.

Aliquot: The small portion of a specimen taken for an assay.

Analyte: A substance or constituent for which a laboratory conducts testing.

Approved State Laboratory Program: A licensure or other regulatory program for laboratories in a state, whose requirements are imposed under state law, that have received HCFA approval based on the state's compliance with 42 CFR Part 493.

Assay: The analysis of the purity of a substance or determination of the amount of any particular constituent in a mixture.

Assignment: An agreement by a provider (physician or supplier) to accept a Medicare beneficiary's rights to benefits under Supplementary Medical Insurance (Part B), to bill the Medicare carrier rather than the patient, and to accept Medicare's approved charge paid by the carrier as payment in full (excluding the beneficiary's 20 percent coinsurance and the deductible). The provider may then bill the beneficiary only for any applicable coinsurance and deductible.

Balance billing: A type of cost sharing under Medicare whereby a beneficiary is responsible for the difference between the physician's submitted charge and the Medicare-allowed charge on unassigned claims, up to a maximum permitted by Medicare.

Beneficiary: An individual entitled to receive Medicare services.

Budget neutrality: Adjustment of payment rates when policies change so that total spending under the new rules is the same as it would have been under the previous payment rules.

Bundling: The use of a single payment for a group of related services.

Capitation payment: A method of paying for medical care by a prospective per capita payment that is independent of the number of services received.

Carrier: An organization that has contracted with DHHS to process and pay approved physician and supplier claims, and perform other services under Medicare Part B.

Case mix: A measure of the mix of cases being treated by a particular health care provider that is intended to reflect the patients' different needs for resources. Case mix is generally established by estimating the relative frequency of various types of patients seen by the provider in question during a given period and may be measured by factors such as diagnosis, severity of illness, utilization of services, and provider characteristics.

Central Statistical Carrier: Mandated by the 1997 BBA, the CSC would be designated from the consolidated regional laboratory carriers to conduct analyses of claims data. This has yet to be implemented.

Charge-based relative value scale: A value scale based on the relationship between current charges for various services.

Chemical hygiene plan: A plan for addressing the specific hazards found in a laboratory and its approach to dealing with them which is required of any laboratory that uses hazardous chemicals.

Clinical Laboratory Improvement Act/Amendments, 1988: Passed in 1967 and amended in 1988, the purpose of CLIA is to ensure the accuracy, reliability, and timeliness of patient test results regardless of where the test is performed. The statute defines a laboratory as any facility that examines human specimens for the diagnosis, prevention, or treatment of any disease or impairment of, or the assessment of the health of, human beings. Any facility that meets this definition must have the appropriate CLIA certificate to perform laboratory tests if it wants to participate in Medicare or Medicaid. To obtain the certificate, state or federal inspectors must survey the laboratory. All suppliers and providers that perform laboratory testing, even if no laboratory per se is part of the facility, must also hold the appropriate valid CLIA certificate and meet applicable CLIA requirements for the testing offered.

CLIA-exempt laboratory: A laboratory that has been licensed or approved by a state where HCFA has determined that the state has enacted laws relating to laboratory requirements that are equal to or more stringent than CLIA requirements and where the state licensure program has been approved by HCFA in accordance with subpart E of 42 CFR Part 493.

Clinical laboratory services: A subset of overall laboratory services, these are tests conducted to diagnose a disease, screen a patient to identify abnormalities, or monitor a patient's condition.

Coinsurance: Also called copayment, the percentage of covered hospital and medical expenses, after subtraction of any deductible, for which an insured person is responsible. Under Medicare Part B, after the annual deductible has been met, Medicare will generally pay 80 percent of approved charges for covered services and supplies; the remaining 20 percent represents the coinsurance, which the beneficiary pays. Laboratory services are currently exempt from coinsurance.

Competitive bidding: A pricing method that elicits information on costs through a bidding process to establish payment rates that reflect the costs of an efficient health plan or health care provider.

Compliance Program Guidance: Revised version of the Model Compliance Plan for Clinical Laboratories, published by the DHHS Office of Inspector General (63 Fed. Reg. 45076, Aug. 24, 1998).

Conversion factor: The multiplier used to translate relative value units into dollar amounts for payments under a fee schedule.

Copayments: Flat fees, typically modest, that insured persons must pay for a particular unit of service, such as an office visit, an emergency room visit, or having a prescription filled. (See coinsurance.)

Cost sharing: The generic term that includes copayments, coinsurance, and deductibles; also, out-of-pocket payments.

Cost shifting: Increasing revenues from some payers to offset losses and lower net payments from other payers.

Cross-walking: When HCFA determines that a new test is sufficiently similar to an existing code, it may assign a National Limitation Amount for payment based on payment data from an existing code.

Current Procedural Terminology code: A code indicating the particular procedure that is performed, based on the Physicians' Current Procedural Terminology, published by the American Medical Association. CPT codes for laboratory services range from 80049 through 89300.

Diagnosis-related groups: Entries in a taxonomy of types of hospitalization based on groupings of diagnostic categories drawn from the International Classification of Diseases and modified by the presence of a surgical procedure, patient age, presence or absence of significant morbidities or complications, and other relevant criteria. DRGs have been mandated for use in establishing payment amounts for individual admissions under Medicare's prospective hospital payment system as required by the Social Security Amendments of 1983 (Public Law 98-21).

Diagnostic test: A test that searches for the presence of an infectious organism, such as a virus or parasite, may find pathology such as cancerous cells, or may help distinguish between different possible causes of a symptom.

DNA marker: A specific gene sequence within a chromosome, indicating the inheritance of a certain trait.

Episode of care: This term is most often used in reference to the monetary costs of an individual's sickness. It includes length of care in special care unit or hospital, nursing care costs in the hospital, professional and technical services, physician services, respiratory services, respiratory therapy, pharmaceuticals, intravenous therapy, collateral diseases, and complications.

Esoteric test: A relatively uncommon test that is often complex and expensive to conduct or depends on specialized interpretative skill. Laboratories that specialize in esoteric testing are usually affiliated with a university or research institution but may also be independent.

Federal Advisory Committee Act: Section 15 of the Federal Advisory Committee Act, signed into law in 1997, clarifies public disclosure requirements that are applicable to the National Academy of Sciences (NAS). Under these amendments, the NAS is required to implement measures that make its processes more accessible to the public while still preserving its independence from government control.

Fee-for-service: A type of plan under which the provider is paid for each service or bundle of services provided.

Fee schedule: A method of paying for medical care that prospectively sets out the fees to be paid for each service provided.

Fiscal intermediary: An organization (usually an insurance company) that has an agreement with HCFA under Medicare Part A to process claims and perform related functions.

Focused medical review: Designed to identify patterns of inappropriate or unnecessary testing, this evaluation could be targeted at particular laboratories and physicians, selected geographic areas, or specific tests that are expected to yield a high return.

Gap-filling: The process of collecting data on the amount that labs are charging in order to establish the payment rate for a new code.

Genetic test: A test that is able to detect a gene mutation, either inherited or caused by the environment.

HCFA Common Procedural Coding System: In popular usage, a national code established by the Health Care Financing Administration. HCPCS include three tiers: Level I consists mainly of CPT codes; Level II, national codes assigned by HCFA; and Level III, codes that are locally assigned.

Health Care Financing Administration: The federal agency within the U.S. Department of Health and Human Services that administers the Medicare and Medicaid programs.

Health maintenance organization: An organization that delivers and manages health services under a risk-based arrangement. The HMO usually receives a monthly premium or capitation payment for each enrollee that is based on a projection of what the typical patient will cost.

Health professional shortage area: An urban or rural geographic area, population group, or public or nonprofit private medical facility that the Secretary of Health and Human Services determines is being served by too few health professionals.

Hospital laboratory: A laboratory located in or operated by a hospital or its organized medical staff.

ICD-9-CM code: A five-digit code indicating a patient's diagnosis that is based on the International Classification of Diseases, Ninth Revision, Clinical Modification. Contractors may require ICD-9 codes as evidence of medical necessity for specific testing.

Independent laboratory: A laboratory that is independent of both an attending and consulting physician's office and a hospital.

Inflation factor: The variable used for updating fee schedules, which Congress determines during the budget reconciliation process. It can be used to reflect changes in the general economy and in the input costs for producing laboratory services.

Laboratory: A facility for the virological, microbiological, serological, chemical, immunohematological, hematological, biophysical, cytological, pathological, or other examination of materials derived from the human body for the purpose of providing information for the diagnosis, prevention, or treatment of any disease or impairment of, or the assessment of the health of, human beings. These examinations also include procedures to determine, measure, or otherwise describe the presence or absence of various substances or organisms in the body. Facilities that only collect or prepare specimens (or both) or only act as a mailing service, and do not perform tests are not considered laboratories.

Local medical review policy: A policy developed by a carrier or fiscal intermediary that establishes the circumstances under which a particular procedure, such as a laboratory test, will be considered medically necessary.

Managed care organization: Any third-party payer that employs cost-control or utilization-control mechanisms to direct the use of health care services.

Medicare Carrier Jurisdiction: One of 56 carrier regions or jurisdictions, each of which is roughly equivalent to a state, with some larger states divided into smaller regions.

Medicare contractor: A commercial insurance company or a Blue Cross/Blue Shield plan that contracts with HCFA to process claims. For Part A providers, contractors are called "fiscal intermediaries;" for Part B providers they are called "carriers."

Medicare Part A: The portion of Medicare that covers services provided by hospitals, skilled nursing facilities, hospices, and some home health services.

Medicare Part B: The portion of Medicare that covers physician services, hospital outpatient services, laboratory services, and others.

Medicare Part C (Medicare+Choice): A new part of Medicare authorized by the Balanced Budget Act of 1997, intended primarily to expand managed-care coverage options for beneficiaries. It replaced the existing system of Medicare risk and cost contracts. It enables beneficiaries to enroll in a coordinated care plan (HMO, PPO), a private fee-for-service plan, or a high-deductible plan with a medical savings account.

Model Compliance Plan: Original version of the guidance for laboratories on compliance issues promulgated in 1997 by the OIG.

Monitoring test: A test that is used to track disease progression or improvement, identify side effects and complications, monitor drug levels, or assess prognosis.

Most favored nation: A title borrowed from the language of international trade. It refers to a system whereby laboratories would provide services to Medicare beneficiaries for the lowest rate they accept from any other payer.

Nanotechnology: The science of building miniature devices out of small particles such as individual atoms, molecules, viruses, or cells.

National Fee Schedule: An idea proposed to replace the 56 current Medicare laboratory fee schedules.

National Limitation Amount: A percentage of the median of all carriers' fees that is used as a cap for Medicare reimbursement.

Negotiated rulemaking: An innovative rulemaking process that brings the government together with interested parties in an attempt to agree on the terms of a proposed rule. Use of this process was mandated by the 1997 BBA to establish uniform coverage, payment, and administrative policies for clinical laboratory services under Medicare Part B.

Outreach testing: Testing conducted in a hospital laboratory for nonhospital patients.

Personal protective equipment: Gear worn by health care workers and laboratory personnel to minimize the transmission of infectious diseases.

Pharmacogenomics: A method of prescribing based on the following: because an individual's genes affect the response to medications, a physician may base prescribing decisions on the patient's genetic makeup.

Phenotype: The physical expression of a trait or characteristic as determined by an individual's genetic makeup, or genotype.

Physician office laboratory: A clinical laboratory in a physician's office.

Point-of-care test: A test conducted by a health professional during a patient encounter. Test results are typically available a few minutes after the specimen is collected.

Polymerase chain reaction: An esoteric test that uses specialized techniques to amplify the amount of DNA in the sample specimen.

Preferred provider organization: An arrangement between a provider network and a health insurer or a self-insured employer. Providers generally accept payments less than the traditional fees-for-service payments in return for a potentially greater share of the patient market.

Prospective payment system: Payment for medical care on the basis of rates established before the period in which they apply. The unit of payment may vary from individual medical services to broader categories, such as hospital case, episode of illness, or person (capitation).

Provider: A facility, clinical laboratory, supplier, or physician who furnishes medical services to beneficiaries.

Pull-through: A situation in which a laboratory undercuts its own pricing structure to win capitated managed care contracts in the hope that participating managed care physicians will also use the laboratory's services for their non-managed care patients.

Reference laboratory: A laboratory that conducts tests for other laboratories; reference laboratories are usually large and may be independent or hospital based.

Reflex test: A test reordered by a physician after an abnormal test result.

Relative value scale: An index that assigns weights to each medical service; the weights represent the relative amount to be paid for each service.

Research test: A test in which specimens are examined for the purpose of understanding a condition better or developing a clinical test.

Resource based relative value scale: A system that bases payment on the relative amount of resources required to provide a service—a common payment method for physicians' services.

Retrospective payment system: One in which the actual payment amount is based on costs or charges and is not known at the time of service.

Screening test: A test that helps a physician find abnormalities, regardless of whether the patient exhibits symptoms.

Sole community hospital: A hospital that is located 25–35 miles from other similar hospitals, serves at least 75 percent of the local residents needing such inpatient care, and meets the detailed criteria contained in 42 C.F.R., Part 412.92.

STAT: Literally, at once. Medically, this refers to tests that are expedited for immediate processing and return of results.

Sustainable growth rate: The target rate of expenditure growth set by the SGR system incorporated in the Medicare fee schedule for physicians.

Sustainable growth rate system: A revision to the volume performance standard system, enacted as part of the BBA of 1997, that serves as the mechanism for setting fee updates for the Medicare fee schedule. It uses a single conversion factor and bases target rates of growth on growth of gross domestic product and other factors.

Technical laboratory personnel: Highly trained or technically certified individuals capable of advanced processing or evaluation of laboratory tests.

Turnaround time: The amount of time that elapses from the initiation of a laboratory test until results from that test are reported to the clinician or patient.

Unbundling: Charging individually for tests that should be billed as a panel at a lower aggregate rate.

Update factor: The year-to-year increase in the Medicare base payment amounts for providers such as PPS hospitals and dialysis facilities and in the target amounts for PPS-excluded hospitals and units.

Venipuncture: Surgical puncture of a vein, generally to draw a blood sample for testing.

Waived test: A laboratory test defined by CLIA standards that can be conducted with minimal chance of error.

This list is based on glossaries included in the following reports:

Health Care Financing Administration. Health Standards and Quality Bureau. 1994. *Laboratory Surveyor Training Manual.* Washington, DC.

Kazon, P.M. 1999. *Doing Business with Medicare: A Policy Guide for Clinical Laboratory Testing,* Washington, DC: Washington G-2 Reports.

U.S. Congress, MedPAC, 1999. *Report to the Congress: Medicare Payment Policy.* Washington, DC: Medicare Payment Advisory Commission.

U.S. Congress, Office of Technology Assessment. 1986. *Payment for Physician Services: Strategies for Medicare.* OTA-H-294. Washington, DC: U.S. Government Printing Office.

APPENDIX A

Acknowledgments

Sue Auxter
American Association of Clinical Chemistry

Kathy Ayers
Clinical Laboratory Management Association

Vickie S. Baselski
University of Tennessee

Mark S. Birenbaum
American Association of Bioanalysts

Melvin C. Bishop
Biological Technology Laboratory, Inc.

Jeffrey Boothe
Oppenheimer Wolff & Donnelly L.L.P.

Tom Bradley
Congressional Budget Office

Geri Brennan
University of Chicago

Mitchell Burken
Health Care Financing Administration

Ted Cartwright
American Society of Clinical Pathologists

Bonnie Bisol Cassidy
CHPS Consulting (Center for Health Policy Studies)

Alan F. Cohen
Physician Office Lab News

Delores Crujeiras
Health Care Financing Administration

Brigid Davison
Health Care Financing Administration

Zachary Dyckman
CHPS Consulting (Center for Health Policy Studies)

Jack Emery
American Medical Association

Joyce Eng
Health Care Financing Administration

Lee Feehely
Health Care Financing Administration

Laurie Feinberg
Health Care Financing Administration

Rodney Forsman
Mayo Reference Services

Joanne Glisson
American Clinical Laboratory Association

Sarah Grantham
CHPS Consulting (Center for Health Policy Studies)

Carl Graziano
CAP Today

Anita Greenberg
Health Care Financing Administration

George Greenberg
Office of the Assistant Secretary for Planning and Evaluation, Department of Health and Human Services

Ellen Griffith
Health Care Financing Administration

George Grob
Office of the Inspector General, Department of Health and Human Services

Thomas Gustafson
Health Care Financing Administration

Joseph Hackett
Food and Drug Administration

Mike Hadad
Aegis Healthcare Solutions

Tzvi Hefter
Health Care Financing Administration

Peter Hickman
Health Care Financing Administration

Lee Hilborne
RAND

Susan Hildebrandt
American Association of Family Physicians

Hugh Hill
Health Care Financing Administration

Tom Hoerger
Research Triangle Institute

Christopher Hogan
Direct Research, L.L.C.

Devery Howerton
Centers for Disease Control and Prevention

Peter Kazon
Mintz Levin

Celeste Kirschner
American Medical Association

Danford R. Layne
Health Care Financing Administration

George T. Linial
Clinical Laboratory Management Association

Brian Loy
AdminaStar

Thomas Marciniak
Consultant

Vic McVicker
Health Care Financing Administration

Ann Meadow
Health Care Financing Administration

Katie Merrell
University of Chicago

Henry Miller
CHPS Consulting (Center for Health Policy Studies)

Peter Oswald
General Accounting Office

Mike Palmer
College of American Pathologists

Elissa Passiment
American Society for Clinical Laboratory Science

Greg Raab
Raab & Associates

Paul A. Raslavicus
College of American Pathologists

Susan Reardon
Johnson and Johnson

Amy Schwartz
Gray Sheet

Jacqueline L. Sheridan
Health Care Financing Administration

Evelyn Soler
Colegio de Tecnologos Medicos de Puerto Rico

Charlie Spalding
Computer Science Corporation

Mary Anne Stevenson
Health Care Financing Administration

Joan Stieber
Health Care Financing Administration

Vince Stine
American Association of Clinical Chemistry

Robin Stombler
American Society of Clinical Pathologists

David Sundwall
American Clinical Laboratory Association

Deborah Thomas
Health Care Financing Administration

Carter Warfield
Health Care Financing Administration

Teresa Waters
Northwestern University

Alice S. Weissfield
Microbiology Specialist Inc.

Dennis Weissman
Washington G-2 Reports

Mary Wiley
Grantmakers In Health

Craig Winslow
General Accounting Office

Mark Wynn
Health Care Financing Administration

APPENDIX B
Medicare Clinical Laboratory Payments: The National Limitation Amount and Its Relationship to Payment Amounts

Katie Merrell
Center for Health Administration Studies, University of Chicago

Under current policy, Medicare payments for ambulatory clinical laboratory services are based on 56 regional fee schedules, subject to a service-specific national limit. Each regional fee schedule is based on charges in 1984, subject to a series of annual reductions and updates since then. The median of these updated base payment rates is calculated for each service to establish the National Limitation Amount (NLA), which is currently set at 74 percent of the median. Actual payment for a particular service in a particular area is then equal to the lesser of the regional base rate and the NLA. This appendix explores the relationships among regional fee schedules, the NLA, and actual payment amounts. By comparing current laboratory payments to the NLA, it provides estimates of the financial implications of an NLA-based national fee schedule.

In 2000, nearly 84 percent of payment amounts (at the region service level) were set at the NLA.[1] This suggests that there is effectively a national fee schedule, where relative service payments are determined by the relationship between median charges in 1984 across the carriers, coupled with gap-filled and cross-walked values for codes established since then.[2]

Analysis of 2000 payment rates reveals that the high prevalence of the NLA in determining payments suppresses the variation in payment amounts across carriers. More than 16 percent of updated base amounts are at least 25 percent less than the median base amount, while more than 21 percent exceed the

[1]The 2000 fee schedules were downloaded from the Health Care Financing Administration's (HCFA) Web page (http://www.hcfa.gov/ stats/pufiles.htm) in February 2000.

[2]Gap-filling and cross-walking are two techniques used by HCFA and its carriers to develop fee schedule values for new services.

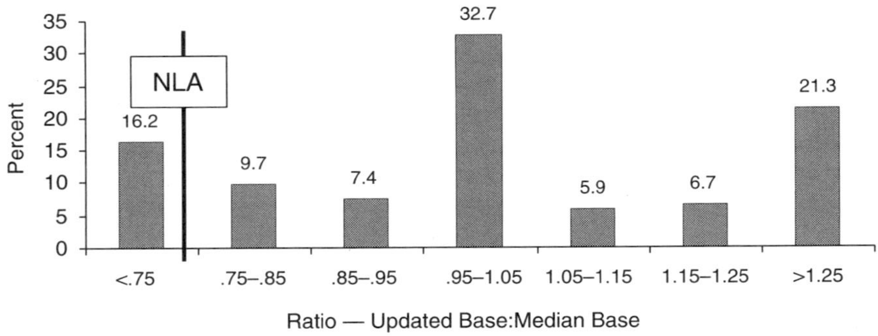

FIGURE B.1 Medicare laboratory fee schedules FY 2000 updated base amounts compared to median base amounts.

median by at least 25 percent (Figure B.1). In other words, nearly 40 percent of the values in carrier fee schedules differ by more than 25 percent from the relevant service median value. Those that fall well below the median will be paid at rates below the NLA, while all of those above 74 percent of the median will be paid at the NLA, reducing the effective geographic differences in payments. The NLA is set at 74 percent of the median, so only 16 percent of service payment amounts are less than the NLA. The base rates, however, exhibit geographic variation not reflected in actual payments. For some, such as non-automated urinalysis (CPT 81000), base amounts are tightly clustered across the regional fee schedules (coefficient of variation = 16 percent), while, for others, such as HIV-1 (CPT 87536), there is considerable spread in base rates (coefficient of variation = 67 percent) (Table B.1). With the exception of the HIV-1 test listed, payment for 20 services studied, which include high-volume Medicare services and others of particular policy interest, is set at the NLA in at least 80 percent of carriers; for three services (digoxin assay, parathormone assay, and Pap cytopathology thin layer preparation), all payments are at the NLA.

The NLA is based on an unweighted median of regional fee schedule amounts. As a result, it is not the median value of actual *payments* for each service since service volumes vary across regions. The median value of actual lab payments for a particular service may be much higher (or lower) than the median used to set the NLA. A simple three-region, three-service example illustrates this (Table B.2).

In this example, all fee schedule values in Regions 2 and 3 exceed the NLA, so all payments in these two regions would be set at the NLA. In Region 1, payments for Services A and B would be set at the regional fee schedule amount while payment for Service C would be capped at the NLA. Overall, 77 percent of payment amounts at the region service level in this hypothetical system would be at the NLA.

TABLE B.1 National Limits and Updated Carrier Base Rates, Selected Laboratory Services

		National Limitation Amount (NLA)		Summary of Updated Carrier Base Rates, 2000					
HCPCS	Brief Description	NLA ($)	% Carrier Payment Amounts @ NLA	Median ($)	Mean ($)	Min ($)	Max ($)	Std. Dev. ($)	Coefficient of Variation
80049	Metabolic panel	11.29	80.36	15.26	16.14	6.34	41.04	5.81	36
80054	Comprehensive metabolic panel	14.61	82.14	19.74	20.45	11.61	33.15	5.57	27
80162	Assay of digoxin	18.35	100.00	24.80	26.15	19.82	48.23	4.80	18
81000	Urinalysis nonauto w/scope	4.37	94.64	5.91	6.11	3.53	8.83	1.00	16
82607	Vitamin B-12	20.83	89.29	28.15	28.75	14.40	77.15	8.81	31
82728	Assay of ferritin	18.83	96.43	25.44	27.13	12.09	49.76	6.31	23
82947	Assay of glucose	5.42	94.64	7.33	7.57	5.18	13.14	1.55	20
83036	Glycated hemoglobin test	13.42	89.29	18.13	18.60	9.66	40.12	5.17	28
83718	Assay of lipoprotein	11.31	91.07	15.29	15.85	7.97	39.47	5.33	34
83970	Assay of parathormone	57.04	100.00	77.08	81.58	57.21	174.87	19.32	24
84154	Assay of PSA free	25.42	94.64	34.35	38.15	20.06	75.64	12.29	32
84443	Assay TSH	23.21	91.07	31.37	31.84	21.74	63.62	6.72	21
85024	Automated hemogram	11.70	76.79	15.81	15.13	8.54	29.69	4.52	30
85025	Automated hemogram	10.74	85.71	14.52	15.03	6.43	29.69	4.45	30
85610	Prothrombin time	5.43	94.64	7.34	7.55	4.39	13.21	1.35	18
86316	Immunoassay	28.76	87.50	38.86	41.53	13.66	104.91	15.60	38
87086	Urine culture/colony count	11.16	89.29	15.08	14.68	5.18	25.08	3.39	23
87536	HIV-1	117.59	76.79	158.91	207.69	67.75	872.10	138.90	67
88142	Cytopathology	0.00	100.00	0.00	0.00	0.00	0.00	0.00	—
88164	Cytopathology TBS	7.15	92.86	9.66	9.61	5.00	14.40	1.96	20

NOTE: Coefficient of variation expresses the standard deviation as a percentage of the mean. Std. Dev. = standard deviation; PSA = prostate specific antigen; TSH = thyroid stimulating hormone; HIV = human immunodeficiency virus; TBS = the Bethesda System.

SOURCE: Analysis of Carrier Fee Schedules and Pricing Amounts for 2000, as reported on the Health Care Financing Administration's Web page.

TABLE B.2 Illustrative Regional Fee Schedules and National Limitation Amounts

	Region 1	Region 2	Region 3	Median	NLA
Service A	$13	$25	$18	$18	$13.32
Service B	$10	$19	$16	$16	$11.84
Service C	$2.60	$3	$3	$3	$2.22

NOTE: The NLA is 74 percent of the median of the regional fee schedule values.

TABLE B.3 Service Volumes

	Region 1	Region 2	Region 3
Service A	100	1,500	1,000
Service B	500	4,500	4,000
Service C	1,000	5,000	4,000

This is not a particularly helpful number, however, because service volumes vary across services and regions. Service C is at the NLA in all three areas, so if it is a high-volume service, the actual number of payments at the NLA would be greater than 77 percent. Similarly, payments in Regions 2 and 3 are all at the NLA, so if they account for more than two-thirds of service volume, the actual number of services paid at the NLA would exceed 77 percent.

Given service volumes, in fact, it would be possible to figure out exactly what percentage of services are paid at the NLA, what share of total spending is at the NLA, and how much more money would be required to pay for all services at the NLA. Based on a set of volumes for the hypothetical system described above (Table B.3), these various measures can be calculated. The resulting estimates indicate the financial implications of an NLA-based fee schedule.

These service volumes imply that, in the hypothetical system, more than 97 percent of service payments would be at the NLA, compared to only 77 percent of regional payment amounts. The share of spending at the NLA would be almost 1 percent lower, because Services A and B, which are not at the NLA in Region 1, account for relatively more spending than volume. In this example, total spending is about 99.4 percent of what it would be if all services were paid at the NLA.[3]

In the case of actual Medicare payments, the simple fact that 84 percent of carrier payment amounts are set at Medicare's NLA does not provide a very accurate estimate of how close current payments are to an NLA-based fee schedule. First, even those services not paid at the NLA may be paid very close to the

[3]Multiplying the payment amounts (the lesser of the fee schedule amount or NLA) in Table B.2 by the volumes in Table B.3 suggests that total spending in this system was $162,440. Multiplying the volumes in Table B.3 by the NLA in Table B.2 shows that if all services were paid at the NLA, then total payments would be $163,392.

NLA. In fact, payment levels not at the NLA average 75 percent of the NLA, across services and carriers. Second, since volumes vary across services and regions, payments for the actual mix of services used by beneficiaries may be closer to (or farther from) the NLA. The ideal way to get a more accurate estimate of how actual payments relate to the NLA would be to use data on service volumes within each carrier to repeat the calculations illustrated above. Unfortunately, reliable service volume data are unavailable at the code-carrier level.

Reasonable estimates can be made, however, based on available data, namely, the distribution of beneficiaries across carriers and of total payments for each lab code. The number of fee-for-service beneficiaries in each carrier area can be used to get some sense of the distribution of service volumes for each code across carriers, although this approach ignores any important regional variation in per capita service use across services.[4] With this distribution, a weighted mean of regional payment amounts can be calculated, which can then be compared with the NLA. The resulting "NLA ratio" tells, in essence, how the mean payment for that service relates to the NLA. In turn, the mean of this service-level NLA ratio, weighted by total spending for each service, would reveal how close total spending is to what would occur under the NLA.

The modified calculation is perhaps most easily illustrated by revisiting the calculations in the above example. Instead of service volumes (Table B.3), imagine that only the distribution of beneficiaries across the three areas and the total spending for each service are available (Table B.4).

A slightly different approach is required to calculate measures such as those reported earlier in the absence of service volumes. First, the distribution of beneficiaries can be used to calculate a service-specific, population-weighted payment amount across the three regions (Table B.5).

The ratio of this amount to the NLA can then be calculated (Table B.5). Finally, the mean of this ratio, weighted by the distribution of total spending (Table B.4), can be calculated. The estimate of 0.992 corresponds well to the earlier estimate that spending was about 99.4 percent of what would occur under the NLA. This alternative approach, although somewhat complicated, appears to allow for developing reasonable estimates without the benefit of service volumes but with the data that are available.

This second approach—population-weighted service-level payment amounts, NLA ratio, and service-level spending-weighted mean of the NLA ratio—can be used with available Medicare data. The distribution of fee-for-service Medicare

---

[4]The appropriateness of using beneficiary counts to summarize payment amounts across carriers was explored through analysis of a subset of services for which credible total volume data were available. For these services, an average payment amount can be calculated by dividing total spending by total service volumes. For this subset of services, the average payment amount was typically within pennies of the beneficiary-weighted average of carrier payment amounts and never differed by more than about 8 percent. This suggests that the use of beneficiary counts to develop service-level payment amounts is appropriate.

beneficiaries across counties is available from the Health Care Financing Administration (HCFA) and can be mapped into the 56 regions underlying the lab fee schedules. Total charge data are available for the 100 codes that accounted for the largest majority of Medicare outpatient lab spending in 1998.[5] Combined, these codes accounted for more than 83 percent of spending, so an analysis of them should be fairly suggestive.[6]

For these top codes, the unweighted service-level NLA ratio across the 56 fee schedules is about 0.98 (compared to about 0.96 for all codes), suggesting that among high-cost or high-volume services, the fee schedule amount is closer to the NLA than for other services. The charge-weighted mean NLA ratio for these services is 0.985, so that across all payments, service payments are about 98.5 percent of the NLA.[7]

TABLE B.4 Population by Region and Spending by Service

	Region 1	Region 2	Region 3	Total Spending
Service A				$34,600
Service B				$105,640
Service C				$22,200
% beneficiaries	7	51	42	

TABLE B.5 Service Payments and NLA Ratio

	Population-Weighted Payment Amount	NLA	Ratio: Weighted Payment Amount to NLA
Service A	$13.30	$13.32	0.998
Service B	$11.70	$11.84	0.988
Service C	$2.22	$2.22	1.000

NOTE: The population-weighted payment amount is calculated from the payment amounts in Table B.2 (minimum of fee schedule amount and NLA) and the population distribution in Table B.4.

---

[5]This analysis is based on 1998 fee schedules, as downloaded from HCFA's Web page (http://www.hcfa.gov/ stats/pufiles.htm) in June 2000, to match the year for which spending data are available.

[6]Several carriers were omitted from this analysis because of problems matching with data on beneficiary counts used for weighting. Similarly, coding discrepancies between data sources limited analyses of the 100 codes with the highest allowed charges to 92 codes. These omissions are unlikely to have important implications for the simple analyses described here.

[7]There is a slight error in this estimate because the total spending weight reflects actual payment levels rather than the NLA. The high correlation between the NLA and the calculated service payment amounts suggests that this error is inconsequential, particularly because spending is used as a weight and not as a measure of absolute levels.

One way to interpret these results is to use them to anticipate the implications of an NLA-based fee schedule. Based on these estimates, an across-the-board NLA reduction of about 1.5 percent would be necessary to create a budget-neutral lab fee schedule based on current NLAs. Conversely, Medicare outpatient lab spending would increase about 1.5 percent if all payments were raised to the NLA.

This estimate is based only on those high-cost or high-volume services that account for most of Medicare spending. The unweighted estimate for all services implies that a reduction of about 4 percent would be necessary, but this is an upper bound that is likely to dramatically overstate the correct amount. Although 1.5 percent is a lower bound, the correct adjustment will lie much closer to 1.5 than to 4 percent, because of the large share of spending accounted for by the services studied. More accurate estimates could be calculated easily from data on total spending for all codes or, better still, service volumes for each code in each region. The present estimates, however, provide fairly strong evidence that Medicare's present payment policy is, in effect, an NLA-based fee schedule.

APPENDIX C
Study of Fees and Payment System Characteristics for Clinical Laboratory Services

Zachary Dyckman, Ph.D.
CHPS Consulting (Center for Health Policy Studies), Columbia, Maryland

EXECUTIVE SUMMARY

The Institute of Medicine (IOM) is conducting a study of Medicare payment methodology for clinical laboratory services. In support of this study, CHPS Consulting (Center for Health Policy Studies) has been asked to conduct a survey of laboratory service payment rates used by different types of health care plans and to compare these payment rates to Medicare payment rates. This information should prove helpful to the IOM both in assessing the existing Medicare payment methodology and fees for clinical laboratory services and in evaluating alternatives for a new payment methodology.

Study Methodology

In February 2000, CHPS conducted a survey of selected Blue Cross/Blue Shield health care plans (payers)[1] regarding payment rates for clinical laboratory services. The surveyed payers offer multiple types of benefit plans, such as indemnity, preferred provider organizations (PPO), point of service (POS), and health maintenance organizations (HMO) plans. A total of 10 payers provided data in response to the survey. The surveyed payers have diverse characteristics and operate in different market settings. The Blue Cross/Blue Shield payers:

---

[1]To avoid confusion, the Blue Cross/Blue Shield plans are referred to as "payers," while the health plans they sponsor (e.g. PPO, HMO) are referred to as "plans."

• serve markets characterized by low, moderate, and high managed care penetration;
• have health insurance market shares ranging from less than 10 to more than 60 percent;
• operate in areas characterized by substantially different population densities and by urban–rural mix;
• operate in all four geographic regions; and
• include for-profit and not-for-profit plans.

The payers were asked to provide current payment rates (fees) for 22 clinical laboratory services, including 21 laboratory tests and venipuncture specimen collection. The selected laboratory services included tests for which Medicare and private payers incur relatively high cost (due to high volume and/or high cost per test), tests of different degrees of complexity, and those that represent different subcategories of laboratory tests. Included in the survey are laboratory services covered under the Medicare laboratory fee schedule as well as anatomic and surgical pathology services that are paid for by Medicare under its fee schedule for physician services.

In addition to requesting data on fees for laboratory services, survey participants were asked to provide descriptions of the primary features of their laboratory payment methodologies as well as capitation rates used for laboratory services under managed care plans.

Study Findings

All of the payers that participated in the clinical laboratory payment survey offered and provided fees used under different types of health plans. The Medicare–private payer fee comparisons were made separately for each benefit plan type.

The primary findings from the clinical laboratory fee comparison are the following:

• Private payer indemnity plan fees are on average 31 percent higher than Medicare fees.
• Private payer PPO and POS plan fees are on average 8 percent higher than Medicare fees.
• Private HMO (non-Medicare, non-Medicaid HMO) fees are on average 2 percent lower than Medicare fees.
• Medicaid HMO fees are on average 12 percent lower than Medicare fees.[2]

Fee comparisons were also made between Medicare and Medicare HMO fees for laboratory services. However, the combination of a small sample of

[2]This finding is based on data from only four Medicaid HMOs and should be treated with some caution.

survey respondents and a possible temporary fee anomaly for one respondent may have caused the results of the Medicare–Medicare HMO fee comparison to be misleading.

Only four payers reported using laboratory service capitation for their managed care programs. The per-member per-month (PMPM) laboratory service capitation rate varies from $0.62 to $0.83.[3]

There are a number of interesting findings relating to characteristics of the private payer PPO plans—the predominant type of private health benefit plan in terms of enrollment—including the following:

- Most health plans require (as does Medicare) that a diagnosis be included with the laboratory claim for it to be approved for payment.
- Unlike Medicare, most health plans allow a physician to bill for tests purchased by the physician from another laboratory.
- There is considerable variation in whether health plans make a separate payment for venipuncture: some do not pay, some pay under all circumstances, and some pay only under specific circumstances—for example, to the physician when another laboratory performs and bills for the test.
- Most health plans use Medicare fees in developing their own laboratory fee structure.
- Some health plans pay higher fees to hospital laboratories than to physicians, and some pay higher fees to physicians than to contracted independent laboratories.

STUDY OBJECTIVES AND DESCRIPTION OF STUDY METHODOLOGY

Background and Study Objectives

The Institute of Medicine of the National Academies is conducting a study of Medicare payment methodology for clinical laboratory services. A primary objective of the study is to assess the strengths and weaknesses of the current Medicare payment methodology for clinical laboratory services. In addition, the study will identify and evaluate alternative payment methodologies that may be considered by Medicare for clinical laboratory services.

One item in the study committee's statement of task is to "investigate and if possible secure and analyze information about costs of performing tests and about payments made by payers other than Medicare." Current Medicare fees for many clinical laboratory tests are based largely on 1983 "prevailing charges," which were imperfect measures of market prices even in 1983.

As part of the IOM study, the Center for Health Policy Studies has been engaged to examine laboratory service payment rates used by different types of

---

[3]For three of the four health plans that use capitation, some laboratory services are not covered under the capitation rate.

health care plans and to compare these to Medicare payment rates. The following are among the questions addressed in this study of comparative laboratory service payment rates:

- Are Medicare fees for clinical laboratory services higher or lower than fees used by private payers?
- How do private payer fees for clinical laboratory services differ among different types of health care plans, such as indemnity plans, PPO plans, POS plans, private HMO plans, Medicare HMO plans, and Medicaid HMO plans?
- What are the characteristics of private payer payment methodologies for clinical laboratory services, including information used in setting fees, documentation requirements for medical necessity, and fee differences among different types of providers?

The following section provides a description of the methodology employed to collect and analyze laboratory payment rates used by payers other than Medicare.

Payment Rate Determination Methodology

The primary objective of the study is to obtain current, valid, and unbiased data on clinical laboratory payment rates used by different types of health plans. A mail and electronic survey with telephone follow-up was conducted of nine private payers that offer multiple types of health plans.[4]

The intent of the payment rate survey was to obtain clinical laboratory payment data for the following types of health benefit plans:

- indemnity plans,
- PPO plans,
- POS plans,
- HMO plans for private (non-Medicare, non-Medicaid) enrollees,
- HMO plans for Medicare enrollees, and
- HMO plans for Medicaid enrollees.

Not all of the surveyed payers offered and provided laboratory payment data for all of the health plan types listed above (see Table C.3). Nine of ten of the surveyed payers provided data for at least three of the health plan types listed above. Data were requested for both fee-for-service and capitation payment methodologies. Data were not sought on payment rates charged by laboratories to physicians. In addition to payment rate data, the survey also included questions relating to characteristics of the clinical laboratory payment systems.

---

[4]A survey of 10 or more payers would have required approval from the Office of Management and Budget, which is a process that could take many months and is beyond the time period for this study.

As an incentive to participate in the survey, payers were told that they would receive comparative fee data, showing how their fees compare to statistical summary fee data for the other surveyed health plans. Also, participants in the survey were provided assurances that their data would be kept strictly confidential and that it would not be possible for anyone to tie data or information provided in response to the survey to specific payers.

Further detail of the clinical laboratory payment survey methodology is provided below.

Selection of Payers

We sought to satisfy several criteria in selecting payers for the laboratory payment survey. The primary criteria were that payers surveyed should:

- offer multiple types of health plans for which we could obtain laboratory fee data (e.g., indemnity, PPO, POS, and HMO plans);
- be representative of different managed care environments (e.g., HMO market concentration of less than 25, 25–50 and, more than 50 percent);
- represent all four geographic regions and different urban and rural settings (e.g., primarily large metropolitan areas, primarily small to midsize metropolitan areas, relatively rural areas);
- have substantial enrollment in non-HMO health plans that use, as does Medicare, contracted provider networks (e.g., PPO plans, managed indemnity plans); and
- include both for-profit and not-for-profit payers.

Based on these criteria, we focused our survey solicitation efforts primarily, but not exclusively, on Blue Cross/Blue Shield plans. Blue Cross/Blue Shield payers were determined to be particularly well suited for this project because they tend to offer a wide variety of health plan types, they use contracted provider networks (as does Medicare) for their PPO and other non-HMO plans, and they serve all geographic regions and all significant health care market areas in the United States.

In February 2000, approximately 25 Blue Cross/Blue Shield payers were sent mail invitations to participate in the clinical laboratory payment survey. In addition four non-Blue Cross/Blue Shield payers were invited to participate. Nine payers, all Blue Cross/Blue Shield plans, agreed to participate in the survey. One of the nine payers subsequently decided not to participate. Two of the eight participating payers own health plans that operate relatively independently in two different markets. Thus, for all practical purposes, 10 health payers participated in this payment survey.

Selected characteristics of the 10 payers are shown in Table C.1. As a group, the participating payers operate in markets with diverse characteristics. Indicators of the survey health payers' diversity include the following:

TABLE C.1 Characteristics of Surveyed Payers

Payers Characteristics	Number of Surveyed Payers
Region	
Northeast	3
South	4
Midwest	2
West	1
Population of Primary Metropolitan Area	
>5 million	2
2–5 million	2
1–2 million	2
<1 million	4
Managed Care (HMO) Concentration[a]	
>50%	2
30–50%	3
20–30%	3
<20%	2
Profit–Nonprofit Status	
For-profit payers	3
Not-for-profit payers	7

[a]In July 1998.

- They have private health insurance market shares of approximately 10 percent–60 percent.
- They serve health care markets that are characterized by different levels of managed care penetration.[5]
- They represent payers in all four geographic regions of the United States.
- They represent payers that serve areas of widely different population sizes and of urban–rural mix.
- They include for-profit and not-for-profit payers.

PPO plans represent the largest benefit plan type for Blue Cross/Blue Shield. This type of health benefit plan is more like the standard Medicare program than other types of private payer benefit plans for the following reasons. Under Medicare and the typical PPO program, enrollees may choose any participating provider and do not have to obtain prior authorization from the plan or from a primary care physician (as under most HMO plans) to see a specialist or to obtain a diagnostic test. Yet, both Medicare and PPO plans typically employ a comprehensive set of medical necessity rules and utilization review protocols. In addition, both Medicare and PPOs (in most markets) rely on relatively large contracted provider networks, and under both programs, contracted providers agree

[5]Based on HMO penetration data as of July 1998 in Interstudy (1999).

not to balance-bill the patient for amounts above the payer-determined fee. (Many indemnity plans do not provide members with balance-billing protection.) Because of the balance-billing restrictions, both Medicare and PPOs have the flexibility to set fee levels below provider charge levels. However both Medicare and PPOs have to be concerned that fees are not set so low that the supply of quality providers willing to serve their enrollees is not adequate.

Selection of Clinical Laboratory Services

The intent, based on initial discussions with IOM project staff, was to collect and conduct a comparative assessment of payment rates (fees) for approximately 20 laboratory tests. These include the 12 tests used in the companion study of laboratory test costs being conducted by CHPS, as well as other laboratory tests. The primary criteria for selection of the additional laboratory tests for the fee survey are that these tests:

- are among the laboratory services with relatively high Medicare payments, because of high volume and/or high per-test cost;
- represent tests of different degrees of complexity and cost, with Medicare national maximum fees ranging from $5 to $175 per test; and
- represent different subcategories of clinical laboratory tests, such as anatomic pathology and surgical pathology, and include tests that are paid under both the Medicare laboratory fee schedule and the Medicare fee schedule for physician services.

The 22 laboratory services for which payment rate data were collected are listed in Table C.2. In addition to laboratory tests, venipuncture, or drawing of specimen, is also included. This procedure is the highest-volume procedure and accounts for the highest aggregate payment of all procedures in the Medicare laboratory fee schedule.

Seventeen of the laboratory services included in the survey are paid for by Medicare under its laboratory fee schedule. Four laboratory tests in our sample, Current Procedural Terminology (CPT) codes 88164, 88305, 88307, and 88342, are classified as anatomic pathology or surgical pathology codes in the American Medical Association (AMA) CPT manual. These procedures are paid for by Medicare under its fee schedule for physician services, which uses the resource-based relative value scale (RBRVS). These procedures are included in the study because it is of interest to determine if the relationship between private payer and Medicare fee levels is similar for laboratory services paid under the Medicare laboratory fee schedule and laboratory services paid under the Medicare RBRVS fee schedule. CPT procedure code 88142 is a newly approved test under Medicare, for which fees (or fee limits) have not yet been determined at the national level. The fee for this procedure is currently determined at the local Medicare carrier level. Four of the tests included in the survey are designated in

TABLE C.2 Laboratory Procedure Codes Included in the Payer Survey

CPT Code	Procedure Description
80049	Basic metabolic panel
80054	Comprehensive metabolic panel
80061	Lipid panel
80092	Thyroid panel with thyroid-stimulating hormone (TSH)
81000	Drug screen; multiple drug classes, each procedure
83036	Hemoglobin; by copper sulfate method, nonautomated, glycated
83970	Parathormone (parathyroid hormone)
84153	Prostate specific antigen (PSA); total
84154	PSA; total, free
84443	TSH
85024	Hemogram and platelet count, automated, and automated partial differential white blood cell (WBC) count (CBC)
85025	Hemogram and platelet count, automated, and automated complete differential WBC count (CBC)
85610	Prothrombin time
86316	Immunoassay for tumor antigen (e.g., cancer antigen 125), each
87086	Culture, bacterial, urine; quantitative, colony count
87536	HIV-1, quantification
88142	Cytopathology, cervical or vaginal (any reporting system), collected in preservative fluid, automated thin layer preparation; manual screening under physician supervision
88164	Cytopathology, slides, cervical or vaginal (the Bethesda system); manual screening under physician supervision
88305	Level IV—surgical pathology, gross and microscopic examination
88307	Level V—surgical pathology, gross and microscopic examination
88342	Immunocytochemistry (including tissue immunoperoxidase), each antibody
G0001/36415	Venipuncture—specimen collection

NOTE: CBC = complete blood count.

the administration's FY 2001 budget to have their national payment limit cut by 30 percent (CPT codes 83036, 84153, 84443, and 87086).

Additional Information Included in the Survey

In addition to fees for specific clinical laboratory services, information relating to the primary characteristics of laboratory payment methodology was requested in the written survey or in follow-up questions addressed to survey respondents. The additional questions related to:

- medical necessity documentation requirements;
- whether payment could be made to a physician or other provider that pays another provider to perform the test;

TABLE C.3 Number of Laboratory Fee Schedules by Benefits Plan Type for the Ten Surveyed Payers

Number of different payers	10
Indemnity fee schedule	11[a]
PPO or POS fee schedule	14[b]
Private HMO fee schedule	9[c]
Medicare HMO fee schedule	4
Medicaid HMO fee schedule	4
Total number of fee schedules	42

[a]10 Indemnity + 1 different independent lab.
[b]10 PPO + 3 different POS + 1 different independent lab.
[c]8 HMO + 1 different POS.

- whether separate payment is made for venipuncture or specimen collection;
- use of Medicare fees as a basis for determining payment rates for laboratory services;
- capitation rates used under HMO and POS plans; and
- Other characteristics of the payment methodology for clinical laboratory services.

A copy of the written survey instrument is provided as Exhibit C.1.

CLINICAL LABORATORY PAYMENT RATES

Introduction

In this section, we report on findings from the survey of clinical laboratory service payment rates. The survey methodology was described earlier. The survey instrument is provided in Exhibit C.1. As indicated earlier, a total of 10 Blue Cross/Blue Shield payers participated in and provided data in response to the laboratory payment survey. These 10 payers serve 10 different markets. Each payer offers, and provided data for, multiple benefit plans (e.g., indemnity, PPO, Medicare HMO). On average, each of the payers provided data for about four different types of benefit plans.

Table C.3 shows the number of different fee schedules that were submitted by the surveyed payers for each type of benefit plan and for which data are included in later tables. Note that where separate fee schedules were submitted for physician laboratory and independent laboratory claims, fees from both fee schedules are included in the fee comparison tables. Thus, ten payers provided fees from indemnity fee schedules, with one payer providing fees from different physician and independent laboratory fee schedules, for a total of eleven indemnity fee schedules.

As discussed in the section "Laboratory Payment System Characteristics," several of the health plans use a single fee schedule for both hospital and other outpatient laboratory providers, while several use a different payment methodology for outpatient clinical laboratory claims submitted by hospital laboratories. Where a separate payment methodology is used for hospital laboratories, payment rates are typically based on discounted charges, incurred hospital costs, or other methodology that results in hospital-specific payment rates. Payment rates under these types of hospital payment methodologies are not included in this study.

PPO and POS plans are considered a single type of benefit plan for fee comparison purposes, and fee data for these plans are reported together in a single table. This is done because, often, there are minimal differences in characteristics between PPO and POS plans, and for most of the survey plans, the same fee schedule is used for both PPO and POS benefit plans. Where a particular health plan uses different fee schedules for PPO and POS plans, fees from both fee schedules are included in the reported data. Thus, data from 14 PPO–POS fee schedules are provided in this report, from 10 PPO fee schedules, 3 POS fee schedules that differ from the PPO fee schedules, and 1 independent laboratory fee schedule that differs from the PPO fee schedule used to pay physicians for laboratory services.

Clinical Laboratory Fee Data

Laboratory procedure fee data are presented in most tables both in dollar values and as a proportion of the Medicare fee in the specific geographic area served by the health plan. In interpreting findings regarding comparative laboratory procedure fee levels, the reader is cautioned to note the number of observations (i.e., the number of benefit plan fee schedules for which data are available for the particular procedure code).

Figure C.1 provides, in bar chart form, summary information on the (unweighted) mean ratio (across procedures and across fee schedules) of health plan fees to Medicare fees for five types of health benefit plans. The ratios are computed without inclusion of the venipuncture procedure (G0001 for Medicare and CPT 36415 for private payers.)

As indicated in the discussion of laboratory service payment systems characteristics, there is considerable variation among private payers as to whether and under what circumstances a separate payment is made for venipuncture. For this reason, we excluded venipuncture from the average fee comparisons shown in Figure C.1.

As expected, Figure C.1 shows that indemnity fees are higher than PPO and POS plan fees, which in turn are higher than private HMO fees. Indemnity and PPO and POS fees are higher than Medicare fees, whereas private HMO fees are lower than Medicare fees. Although Medicare HMO fees appear to be comparable to PPO and POS fees and higher than private HMO fees according to Figure C.1, this may be an aberration due, in part, to only four health plans reporting

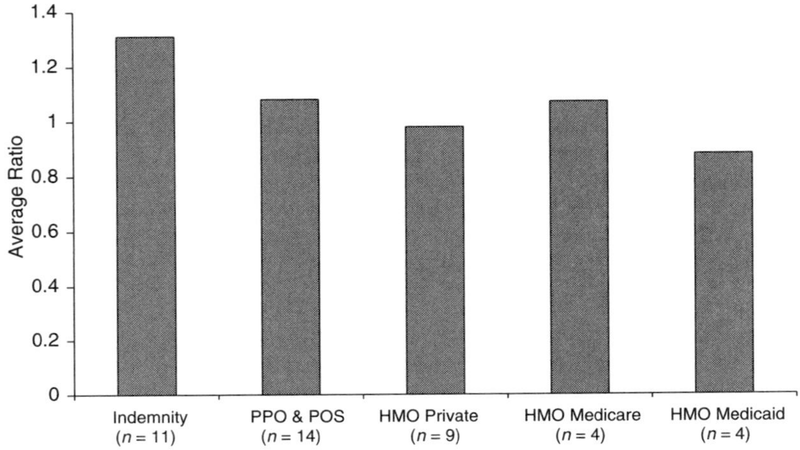

FIGURE C.1 Average (mean) ratio of private payer fees to Medicare fees, 2000.

Medicare HMO fees. This is discussed further below. Medicaid HMO fees are the lowest among fees for the five categories of health plans.

Tables C.4 through Table C.8 provide comparative laboratory fee data for each type of health plan. Shown in these tables are various statistics along with the average (mean) ratio of health plan fee to the local area Medicare fee for each of the individual laboratory procedure codes in our sample. All reported means are simple means, not weighted by claims volume or by health plan enrollment. Also shown in these tables for each procedure is the National Limitation Amount (NLA) of the Medicare laboratory fee schedule, which is the maximum fee that can be paid in any locality under this fee schedule. For procedures covered under the Medicare fee schedule for physician services, the fee shown in the NLA column is the maximum Medicare fee among all of the localities represented by the survey health plans.

The average ratio of the health plan fee to the Medicare fee in the health plan's service area is shown in the last column of Table C.4. Thus, for CPT code 80049, 1.41 represents the average (mean) of the 11 ratios of indemnity plan fee to local Medicare fee for this code. The last row, last column shows the average across procedure codes of these ratios, inclusive and exclusive of the venipuncture procedure (G0001/36415).[6] Indemnity health plan fees are shown in Table C.4.

[6]Based on reported 1998 Medicare claims expenditures, Medicare spending for venipuncture is approximately 4 percent of total outpatient clinical laboratory costs. The venipuncture code has slightly less than a 5 percent weight within our laboratory procedure survey (1 of 21 codes), so the reported differences between the average private payer to Medicare fee ratio with and without venipuncture (1.36 and 1.31) is a close approximation of the true Medicare expenditure weighted difference.

There is considerable variation between the high and low fees among indemnity plans, with the high fee typically eight to ten times higher than the low fee.

The very large indemnity plan fee variation reflects, to a large extent, one indemnity plan using fees based on usual, customary, and reasonable (UCR) charges. Under this plan, the provider has not agreed not to balance-bill the patient for charges in excess of the payer fee. All of the other indemnity plans in the study survey use fee schedules (lower than UCR fees) under provider contracts where the providers have agreed to accept the health plan fee as payment in full, including any required copayments. UCR indemnity plans, although no longer very common, are more prevalent among indemnity plans offered by private health insurance companies (not included among survey plans) than among Blue Cross/Blue Shield plans.

The last rows in Table C.4 show the average ratio of plan fee to Medicare fee, with and without the venipuncture or specimen collection code. As noted above, and discussed in more detail below, some plans pay separately for venipuncture, while others do not. The average ratio of indemnity fee to Medicare fees across all procedures is 1.36 inclusive of test fees that include venipuncture and 1.31 exclusive of test fees that include venipuncture.

In focusing on the average health plan fee to Medicare fee ratios shown in the last column of Table C.4, most ratios are in a relatively narrow range of 1.20 to 1.45, indicating that, on average, indemnity fees are typically 20 to 45 percent higher than area Medicare fees. There is greater variation among the surgical and anatomical procedures paid under the Medicare fee schedule for physician services. For these procedures, the average fee ratio varies from 0.87 to 2.17 among the four procedures for which Medicare fees are available. The average fee ratio for venipuncture among the health plans that pay for this procedure is 2.27.

Table C.5 provides comparative laboratory fee data for PPO and POS plans. This category of health plans represents the largest enrollment among the different types of health benefit plans, for both the United States as a whole and the health plans included in the CHPS survey. It is reported that for those enrolled under employee health benefit plans, 1998 PPO and POS plan enrollment was 98 million while HMO enrollment (not including POS plans) was 59 million in 1998 (Preferred Provider Organization Report, 2000).

For most of the payers that operate both PPO and POS plans, fees are identical for both types, although several use lower fees for POS than for PPO plans. Data for 14 different PPO and POS fee schedules are reported in Table C.5. As indicated above, fees for both a PPO and a POS benefit plan from the same health plan are included in Table C.5 if each type benefit plan uses a different fee schedule.

There is considerable fee variation among different PPO and POS plans, although less so than among indemnity plans. For most laboratory procedure codes, the high fee is two to four times greater than the low fee among the 14 fee schedules.

TABLE C.4 Comparative Indemnity Plan Fees for Selected Clinical Laboratory Services, 2000

			Indemnity Plans				Avg. Ratio of
CPT Code	No. of Obs.	Medicare NLA Fee ($)	Low Fee ($)	High Fee ($)	Median Fee ($)	Mean Fee ($)	Fee to Area Medicare Fee
80049	11	11.29	4.93	49.00	13.00	15.83	1.41
80054	11	14.61	8.06	55.00	14.25	17.95	1.25
80061	11	18.51	10.60	70.00	20.25	23.79	1.32
80092	11	41.66	13.64	125.00	48.00	52.95	1.27
81000	11	4.37	3.04	21.00	5.00	6.84	1.56
83036	11	13.42	7.55	52.00	15.50	17.91	1.34
83970	11	57.04	42.00	150.00	62.74	68.82	1.21
84153	11	25.42	17.19	85.00	29.25	33.60	1.32
84154	10	25.42	17.03	100.00	27.96	35.18	1.38
84443	11	23.21	10.08	88.00	26.75	29.89	1.29
85024	11	11.70	3.60	37.00	12.87	13.50	1.21
85025	11	10.74	3.60	37.00	12.25	12.96	1.21
85610	11	5.43	3.99	26.00	6.25	7.76	1.45
86316	11	28.76	17.55	102.00	31.64	35.73	1.24
87086	11	11.16	6.53	46.00	12.75	14.94	1.34
87536	8	117.59	18.32	410.00	175.00	151.92	1.34
88142	9	N/A	5.21	65.00	25.30	29.75	N/A
88164*	11	14.60	5.21	39.00	9.00	12.70	0.87
88305*	11	86.71	30.81	240.00	74.00	88.08	1.12
88307*	11	175.27	68.00	300.00	117.00	140.40	0.90
88342*	11	44.52	54.58	150.00	67.00	81.63	2.17
G0001/36415*	7	3.00	3.00	15.00	5.00	6.82	2.27
Average ratio with G0001							1.36
Average ratio without G0001							1.31

N/A = National Medicare fee is not yet available for this code.

*Medicare pays for procedure based on the Medicare Fee schedule for physician services.

TABLE C.5 Comparative PPO and POS Plan Fees for Selected Clinical Laboratory Services, 2000

			PPO and POS Plans				Avg. Ratio of
CPT Code	No. of Obs.	Medicare NLA Fee ($)	Low Fee ($)	High Fee ($)	Median Fee ($)	Mean Fee ($)	Fee to Area Medicare Fee
80049	14	11.29	4.93	19.00	12.25	11.65	1.04
80054	14	14.61	5.70	23.00	14.38	13.54	0.97
80061	14	18.51	10.60	30.00	18.38	18.59	1.03
80092	14	41.66	13.64	67.00	45.00	42.87	1.05
81000	14	4.37	3.04	10.75	5.00	5.19	1.19
83036	14	13.42	7.55	21.00	14.25	14.04	1.06
83970	14	57.04	42.00	91.00	61.50	61.41	1.08
84153	14	25.42	19.00	41.00	29.63	28.33	1.11
84154	13	25.42	19.00	41.00	29.25	28.45	1.12
84443	14	23.21	10.08	37.00	24.00	23.40	1.03
85024	14	11.70	3.60	19.00	12.54	11.37	1.03
85025	14	10.74	3.60	17.00	11.50	10.53	1.00
85610	14	5.43	3.87	8.00	6.00	5.66	1.06
86316	14	28.76	17.55	46.00	29.50	29.67	1.05
87086	14	11.16	6.53	18.00	11.88	11.58	1.07
87536	11	117.59	18.32	210.00	150.00	115.26	1.40
88142	12	N/A	5.21	45.00	19.00	25.52	N/A
88164*	14	14.60	5.21	14.00	9.00	9.87	0.70
88305*	14	86.71	30.81	101.00	74.00	73.76	0.97
88307*	14	175.27	68.00	176.00	125.00	126.83	0.85
88342*	14	44.52	51.67	83.00	63.16	71.44	1.87
G0001/36415*	10	3.00	3.00	15.00	5.25	7.25	2.35
Average ratio with G0001							1.14
Average ratio without G0001							1.08

N/A = National Medicare fee is not yet available for this code.

*Medicare pays for procedure based on the Medicare Fee schedule for physician services.

Similar to the indemnity plan fee data, the average PPO and POS to Medicare fee ratio is within a relatively narrow range for most laboratory procedure codes, ranging from 1.00 to 1.12. Variation in this ratio is greatest among the anatomical and surgical pathology codes that are paid for by Medicare under its fee schedule for physician services.

The average ratio of PPO or POS plan fee to Medicare fee across all procedure codes is 1.08 (excluding venipuncture). Thus, PPO and POS laboratory fees (unweighted by volume) are 8 percent higher than Medicare fees. It was noted with reference to comparative fee data in both Tables C.4 and C.5 that there is less variation in the ratio of private health plan fee to Medicare fee for laboratory procedures that are included in Medicare's laboratory fee schedule than for those that are included in its RBRVS fee schedule. One possible explanation for this is that many private payers set their laboratories' fees as a fixed proportion of fees in the Medicare laboratory fee schedule (see "Laboratory Payment System Characteristics), while it is hypothesized, that many payers use the Medicare RBRVS fee schedule in a less structured way. If this hypothesis is correct, less variation can be expected in the private payer to Medicare fee ratio among procedures that are included in the Medicare laboratory fee schedule than among those that are not.

It was noted earlier that four laboratory procedure codes were designated in the administration's FY 2001 budget to have their national payment limit reduced by 30 percent. These codes are shown below, along with the average ratio of PPO and POS plan fee to Medicare fee:

Code	Ratio
83036	1.06
84153	1.11
84443	1.03
87086	1.07

The ratios of PPO or POS plan fee to Medicare fee for these four codes are on average very close to the ratio for all laboratory test procedures (1.07 versus 1.08).

Table C.6 provides data for private HMO plans. On average, private HMO fees are very close to Medicare fees. For most procedure codes, the average ratio of private HMO to Medicare fee is within a range of 0.94 to 1.09. As with indemnity and PPO or POS benefit plans, variation in the average fee ratio is greatest for the anatomical and surgical pathology codes. Across all procedure codes, the average private HMO to Medicare fee ratio is 0.98 (1.01 including venipuncture).

Table C.7 provides fee data for four Medicare HMO plans. Only four of the ten payers that participated in the survey provided fee data for Medicare HMO plans. Because of the limited number of fee schedules and also because one of the four health plans pays higher fees under its private and Medicare HMO plans than it does under its non-managed care plans, the average Medicare HMO to

TABLE C.6 Comparative Private HMO Plan Fees for Selected Clinical Laboratory Services, 2000

		Medicare	Private HMO Plans				Avg. Ratio of Fee to Area
CPT Code	No. Obs.	NLA Fee ($)	Low Fee ($)	High Fee ($)	Median Fee ($)	Mean Fee ($)	Medicare Fee
80049	9	11.29	4.93	22.98	11.29	10.93	0.97
80054	9	14.61	5.70	36.76	13.00	13.83	0.97
80061	9	18.51	10.60	31.43	18.25	17.64	1.01
80092	9	41.66	13.64	54.59	42.00	39.06	0.94
81000	9	4.37	3.04	10.75	4.00	4.77	1.09
83036	9	13.42	7.55	19.85	13.00	12.86	0.97
83970	9	57.04	42.00	86.85	57.00	56.68	0.99
84153	9	25.42	18.69	41.36	26.69	27.64	1.09
84154	8	25.42	17.03	30.00	26.35	25.80	1.01
84443	9	23.21	10.08	33.20	19.00	20.40	0.88
85024	9	11.70	3.60	15.71	10.00	9.15	0.83
85025	9	10.74	3.60	14.24	10.00	8.72	0.82
85610	9	5.43	3.87	6.62	5.00	5.12	0.96
86316	9	28.76	17.55	49.63	27.00	27.83	0.97
87086	9	11.16	6.53	16.54	11.00	10.37	0.93
87536	7	117.59	18.32	175.00	150.00	111.26	1.00
88142	7	N/A	5.21	23.00	14.00	14.60	N/A
88164*	9	14.60	5.21	12.00	8.94	9.18	0.63
88305*	9	86.71	30.81	91.00	64.00	64.73	0.85
88307*	9	175.27	68.00	158.25	108.75	109.69	0.72
88342*	9	44.52	45.00	158.66	56.52	69.47	1.91
G0001/36415*	6	3.00	3.00	10.00	4.05	5.02	1.67
Average ratio with G0001							1.01
Average ratio without G0001							0.98

N/A: National Medicare fee is not yet available for this code.

*Medicare pays for procedure based on the Medicare Fee schedule for physician services.

TABLE C.7 Comparative Medicare HMO Plan Fees for Selected Clinical Laboratory Services, 2000

			Medicare HMO Plans				
CPT Code	No. Obs.	Medicare NLA Fee ($)	Low Fee ($)	High Fee ($)	Median Fee ($)	Mean Fee ($)	Avg. Ratio of Fee to Area Medicare Fee
80049	4	11.29	4.93	22.98	12.65	13.30	1.18
80054	4	14.61	8.06	36.76	13.00	17.71	1.26
80061	4	18.51	12.63	31.43	18.50	20.27	1.22
80092	4	41.66	13.64	54.59	41.50	37.81	0.91
81000	4	4.37	3.04	5.79	5.00	4.71	1.08
83036	4	13.42	7.55	19.85	13.50	13.60	1.03
83970	4	57.04	48.76	86.85	63.50	65.65	1.15
84153	4	25.42	21.77	41.36	30.00	30.78	1.21
84154	3	25.42	17.03	30.00	25.70	24.24	0.95
84443	4	23.21	10.08	33.20	23.50	22.57	0.97
85024	4	11.70	3.90	15.71	11.00	10.40	0.92
85025	4	10.74	3.79	14.24	10.00	9.51	0.89
85610	4	5.43	3.99	6.62	6.00	5.65	1.06
86316	4	28.76	21.77	49.63	29.50	32.60	1.13
87086	4	11.16	6.53	16.54	10.50	11.02	0.99
87536	4	117.59	18.32	175.00	96.25	96.46	0.88
88142	4	N/A	5.21	59.00	18.39	25.25	N/A
88164*	4	14.60	5.21	14.00	9.53	9.57	0.66
88305*	4	86.71	30.81	84.00	66.89	62.15	0.80
88307*	4	175.27	68.00	147.00	112.65	110.08	0.71
88342*	4	44.52	52.78	158.66	66.00	85.86	2.33
G0001/36415*	3	3.00	3.00	12.00	4.60	6.53	2.18
Average ratio with G0001							1.12
Average ratio without G0001							1.07

N/A: National Medicare fee is not yet available for this code.

*Medicare pays for procedure based on the Medicare Fee schedule for physician services.

TABLE C.8 Comparative Medicaid HMO Plan Fees for Selected Clinical Laboratory Services, 2000

		Medicare	Medicaid HMO Plans				Avg. Ratio of Fee to Area
CPT Code	No. Obs.	NLA Fee ($)	Low Fee ($)	High Fee ($)	Median Fee	Mean Fee	Medicare Fee
80049	4	11.29	4.93	12.00	11.27	9.87	0.88
80054	4	14.61	8.06	13.00	11.73	11.13	0.81
80061	4	18.51	12.63	19.00	14.60	15.21	0.92
80092	4	41.66	13.64	44.00	37.28	33.05	0.79
81000	4	4.37	3.04	5.00	4.00	4.01	0.92
83036	4	13.42	7.55	14.00	11.25	11.01	0.83
83970	4	57.04	48.76	59.00	57.50	55.69	0.98
84153	4	25.42	21.77	30.00	26.00	25.94	1.02
84154	3	25.42	17.03	26.00	26.00	23.01	0.91
84443	4	23.21	10.08	24.00	20.50	18.77	0.81
85024	4	11.70	3.90	12.00	7.00	7.48	0.67
85025	4	10.74	3.79	12.00	9.35	8.62	0.81
85610	4	5.43	3.99	6.00	5.00	5.00	0.93
86316	4	28.76	21.77	30.00	26.85	26.37	0.92
87086	4	11.16	6.53	11.00	9.50	9.13	0.82
87536	4	117.59	18.32	175.00	68.13	82.39	0.73
88142	4	N/A	5.21	28.20	13.00	14.85	N/A
88164*	4	14.60	5.21	14.00	7.05	8.33	0.57
88305*	4	86.71	30.81	84.00	51.00	54.20	0.71
88307*	4	175.27	54.00	147.00	89.00	94.75	0.62
88342*	4	44.52	15.00	158.66	61.50	74.17	2.04
G0001/36415*	3	3.00	1.50	10.00	3.00	4.83	1.61
Average ratio with G0001							0.92
Average ratio without G0001							0.88

N/A: National Medicare fee is not yet available for this code.

*Medicare pays for procedure based on the Medicare Fee schedule for physician services.

Medicare ratios should not be considered reliable.[7] The average fee ratio among the four Medicare HMO plans, across all procedures, is 1.07 (1.12 including venipuncture).

Table C.8 provides fee data for Medicaid HMO plans, reflecting the experience of four such plans. On average, Medicaid HMO fees are 12 percent lower than Medicare fees (8 percent including venipuncture).

Summary data for each of the health plans that participated in the survey are provided in Table C.9. Shown in Table C.9, separately for each payer and—within payer—for each benefit plan type, is the average ratio (across procedures) of benefit plan fee to Medicare fee.[8] Of interest is the pattern of fee variation within benefit plan type among the different payers. Also of interest is the fact that a majority of payers use the same fee schedule for different benefit plan types. Some payers use the same fee schedule for all of their benefit plans (Plans C, I, and J), whereas others use the same fee schedule for some but not all of their benefit plans (Plans B, D, F, and H). Some payers face unique contractual, regulatory, or other factors that can affect their fees under specific benefit plans. For example, payer B currently uses a higher fee schedule for its private and Medicare HMO plans than for its indemnity, PPO, and POS plans as a result of a temporary regulatory constraint on adjusting fees. This situation, we are told, is changing and HMO laboratory fees will be reduced in the near future.

Clinical Laboratory Capitation Data

The surveyed payers were asked to provide clinical laboratory service capitation payment data for their managed care plans in addition to fee data. Four of the ten payers that responded to the survey indicated that they use capitation for clinical laboratory services for at least one of their benefit plans. These health plans provided PMPM capitation rates. Table C.10 lists the rates and other characteristics of the capitation programs used by the four health plans.

The average capitation rate among the four health plans is $0.74. This is reasonably close to the $0.81 average PMPM clinical laboratory service capitation rate cited by Klipp (2000), based on a national survey of 700 HMOs in the fall of 1998. The reported PMPM clinical laboratory capitation rates in our sur-

---

[7]CHPS has been told by payment system staff at this Blue Cross/Blue Shield plan that the relatively high Medicare HMO fee is a temporary anomaly that will be changed shortly.

[8]The ratios shown in Table C.9 do not include venipuncture. Also, the average ratios by benefit plan type (shown at the bottom of the table) are slightly different from those shown in Tables C.4 through C.8. This is due to the combined effects of (1) computing the average ratio across health plans in Table C.9 and computing the average ratios across procedures in Tables C.4 through C.8, and (2) missing fee data for some procedures, resulting in a different weighting of fee ratios between the two calculation approaches.

TABLE C.9 Average Ratio of Private Payer Fees to Medicare Fees Across Different Benefit Plans

Plan	Indemnity/ Medicare	PPO/ Medicare	POS/ Medicare	HMO/ Medicare	HMO Medicare/ Medicare	HMO Medicaid/ Medicare
A	1.21	1.08		0.94		
B	1.11	1.00	1.00	1.42	1.42	0.80
C	0.91	0.91				
D	1.57	1.57	1.31	1.01		
E	3.54	1.37	0.86			
F1*	1.06	0.71	0.71	0.71		
F2*	0.73	0.67	0.67	0.67		
G	0.73	0.73	0.73	0.73	0.73	0.73
H	1.08	1.08	1.06	0.95	1.06	0.95
I	1.00	1.00	1.00	1.00	1.00	1.00
J	1.21	1.21	1.21	1.21		
Average	1.29	1.03	0.95	0.96	1.05	0.87

*Plan F submitted separate laboratory fee data for physicians and independent laboratories.

TABLE C.10 Characteristics of Clinical Laboratory Service Capitation Programs, 2000

Benefit Plans	PMPM Capitation Rate ($)	Excluded Clinical Laboratory Services
POS plan	0.83	Surgical pathology
POS, private HMO, Medicare HMO	0.76	None
Private HMO	0.62	Cytology, histology
Private HMO	0.73	Urinalysis, complete blood count

vey are each less than 1 percent of typical HMO PMPM premiums for all medical services of $120–$150.[9]

The four health plans that reported use of laboratory service capitation have diverse characteristics. They operate in highly urbanized and less urbanized environments, in markets with significantly different degrees of managed care plan penetration, and in three of the four geographic regions of the United States.

Comparison of Fees

It is of interest to compare the clinical laboratory fee data obtained in this study with current fee data from other sources. We identified one published source of relatively current fee data for clinical laboratory services. *Lab Industry Strategic Outlook,* published by Washington G-2 Reports, provides 1999 data on "managed care" fees for 20 laboratories in five cities based on payer fee surveys conducted by Caredata (Klipp, 2000). G-2 Reports provides three fees for each of the 20 procedure codes—high, typical, and low.

Four of the G-2 Reports procedure codes match procedure codes included in this survey, and two of the five cities in the G-2 Reports are in market areas represented by the Blue Cross/Blue Shield payers in this survey. We compared the 2000 CHPS PPO and POS fees with the 1999 G-2 Reports fees for the four procedures in the two cities. The following summarizes the results of the 12 fee comparison:[10]

- for 10 of 12 fees, the CHPS fee was within G-2 Reports' low to high range; and

[9]The range of HMO premiums of $120 to $150 for 2000 is based on a 1999 CHPS analysis of HMO premiums updated to 2000 and a review of estimated premiums from alternative health industry sources.

[10]There are three PPO and POS fee schedules in the two cities, resulting in 12 procedure fee comparisons.

• for 8 of 12 fees, the CHPS fee was closer to the "typical" fee reported by G-2 Reports than to the low or high fee.

Based on the limited comparison of the CHPS survey fee data and the fee data included in G-2 Reports, the CHPS survey fees are certainly consistent with other fee survey data. Medicare fees fall within the range of fee schedules reported in the CHPS survey.

It was noted earlier that all of the private payers that participated in this survey are Blue Cross/Blue Shield payers. CHPS' experience with Blue Cross/Blue Shield payers, as well as with other payers, indicates that there is considerable variation among localities in whether the Blue Cross/Blue Shield payers are among the lower payers, or the higher payers, to providers. Although this cannot be proved without considerably more research, it is the author's view that the payer fee data reported in this study are not substantially different than aggregate payer experience for the indemnity, PPO and POS, and private HMO benefit plans.

CHARACTERISTICS OF LABORATORY SERVICE PAYMENT SYSTEMS

Survey Approach

In addition to comparative payment data, payers were also asked to provide information relating to characteristics of their provider payment systems. This information was obtained via responses to the written payer survey attached as Exhibit C.1, as well as responses to subsequent questions addressed to survey participants.

We are highly confident that accurate descriptions of payment characteristics were obtained for the payers' PPO benefit plans, based on the written responses to the surveys as well as additional information provided in subsequent telephone and e-mail follow-up communications. For most of the survey payers, much if not all of the payment system features used for PPO programs are also applicable to the health plans' indemnity and POS benefit plans.

Laboratory Payment System Characteristics

Table C.11 summarizes payment system characteristics for PPO benefit plans. For most health plans, this information would be similar for all of their benefit plans that pay for laboratory services based on fee for service, specifically, their indemnity, POS, and to some extent, HMO plans.[11]

The first row of Table C.11 addresses the issue of whether the health plan requires that a diagnosis be provided on the claim for clinical laboratory service

[11]Payment system characteristics are provided in Table C.11 for nine health plans that reported useful data.

in order for the claim to be paid. Although all health plans request diagnosis codes on their laboratory claims, two of the nine plans will pay the claim if diagnosis is missing.

The second issue addressed in Table C.11 is whether there are some clinical laboratory tests for which payment will not be made by the plan unless one or more specific diagnoses appear on the claim. Four of the nine health plans require specific diagnoses in order to approve coverage for selected laboratory tests.

Medicare and Medicaid do not allow payment to a provider for a laboratory test unless the provider has actually performed the test. In addition, several states have enacted laws imposing a similar payment restriction that is applicable to private payers. Thus, under Medicare, Medicaid, and private insurance and self-pay situations in a minority of states, a physician cannot bill for a test that is sent out to be performed by an independent laboratory. Two-thirds of the reporting health plans allow payment to the physician for tests that the physician purchases from other providers, regardless of the price paid by the physician for the tests.

The fourth row in Table C.11 addresses whether the health plan makes a separate payment for venipuncture, in addition to paying for the test itself and for an office visit (if it occurs). Payment for venipuncture varies across the plans. Two health plans allow payment for venipuncture under all circumstances; two plans never allow it; four plans allow payment only when the provider is not also billing for the test; and one plan allows payment only in the physician office setting but not in the independent or hospital laboratory setting.

In the previous chapter, we have noted that for most PPO and POS plans, the relative fee structure among the laboratory procedure codes that are covered under the Medicare laboratory fee schedule is very similar to Medicare's relative fee structure. It turns out that this is no coincidence. Six of the nine health plans report that they use Medicare fees as a basis for setting their own fees for a significant portion of their laboratory services. However, these health plans' fees may be set at a specific percentage above or below Medicare fees, and the fees may not be updated when Medicare fees are updated.

The next issue relates to whether the health plans use different fee schedules for laboratory service claims submitted by physicians and by independent laboratories. Five of the nine health plans use the same fee schedule for both physicians and independent laboratories. The remaining four health plans pay lower fees to at least some independent laboratories (not necessarily all) with whom they have contracts than they do to physicians.

The fee comparison tables provided earlier include separate independent laboratory fee schedules for only one health plan. This health plan, which operates in a state that does not allow payment for laboratory tests to a provider that has not performed the test, is the only health plan that submitted separate independent laboratory fee schedule data. The lack of inclusion in the fee comparison tables of additional independent laboratory fee data for other health plans that use a separate laboratory fee schedule may result in an upward bias in the reported health plan fees. However, this bias may be small since, based on previous analyses performed for Blue Cross/Blue Shield plans, most payments for laboratory services made by health plans that allow payments to physicians for tests performed by independent laboratories, are made to the physicians.

The last issue addressed in Table C.11 is whether health plans pay higher fees to hospital laboratories than they do to physicians. Five of the nine health plans pay hospitals different fees (typically, higher fees) for outpatient tests than the fees paid to physicians. For most of these health plans, payments are based on a cost reimbursement formula, on discounted hospital charges, or on special fee arrangements negotiated with specific hospitals. The fee comparison tables (Tables C.4–C.8) do not include any of these special fee arrangements for laboratory tests provided by hospital laboratories.

REFERENCES

Interstudy. 1999. Competitive Edge, Part III: Regional Market Analysis, Interstudy.

Klipp, J. 2000. *Lab Industry Strategic Outlook 2000: Market Trends and Analysis*, Washington, DC: Washington G-2 Reports.

Preferred Provider Organization Report: 1999 Edition. 2000. Chicago: American Association of Preferred Provider Associations.

Continued

TABLE C.11 Summary of Laboratory Service Payment System Characteristics for PPO Plans, 2000

Payment System Characteristics	Health Plan A	Health Plan B	Health Plan C	Health Plan D	Health Plan E	Health Plan F	Health Plan G	Health Plan H	Health Plan I
Requires diagnosis for payment of claim	Yes	Yes	No	Yes	Yes	Yes	Yes	No	Yes
Requires specific diagnosis for payment for selected tests	No	No	Yes	Yes	No	No	No	Yes	Yes
Allows physician to bill for test performed by another lab	Yes	Yes	Yes	Yes	Yes	No	No	Yes	No
Pays separately for venipuncture (G0001/36415)	No[a]	No[a]	No	Yes	Yes	Yes[b]	No	No[a]	No[a]
Fee schedule based on Medicare fees	No	Yes	Yes	Yes	Yes	No	No	Yes	Yes
Pays higher fees to physicians than to independent labs	No	No	No	No	Yes	Yes	Yes	No	Yes[c]
Pays higher fees to hospital than to physicians	Yes	Yes	No	Yes	No	Yes	No	Yes	No

[a]Payment is not made for venipuncture to a provider that submits a claim for the laboratory tests. Payment is made to a physician if another provider submits a claim for tests.
[b]Venipuncture is paid for only in the physician office setting, regardless of whether the physician performs the test or it is sent out to an independent or hospital laboratory.
[c]As of December 1, 2000, the same fee schedule will be used for all laboratory types.

EXHIBIT C.1: SURVEY INSTRUMENT FOR STUDY OF PAYMENT RATES FOR LABORATORY SERVICES

All information and data provided in this survey will be kept strictly confidential, within CHPS Consulting including the identification of health plans participating in the survey.

If you have any questions regarding this survey, please contact Zach Dyckman, Project Director, at:

Phone: (410) 715-9400 x320
Fax: (410) 715-9718
E-mail: zdyckman@chpsconsulting.com

Please return the completed form on or before March 25, 2000.

Dr. Zachary Dyckman
The Center for Health Policy Studies
10440 Little Patuxent Parkway, 10th Floor
Columbia, MD 21044

Responses to questions and payment data can be provided on this survey form, on separate pages, or through E-mail. If you use E-mail, please print out and return a copy of your responses to Dr. Dyckman, via Fax or mail.

Thank You

Section I. Background and General Description of Laboratory Payment Methodologies

1. Name of Health Plan: ________________________________

2. Individual primarily responsible for completing survey:
   Name and title________________________________
   Phone ____________________FAX ________________________
   E-mail address________________________________

3. Briefly describe the laboratory payment methodology used by each of your different types of benefit plans, e.g., indemnity, PPO, POS, HMO (private), HMO (Medicare, Medicaid), etc. Indicate whether you use a fee schedule, negotiated fees, discount on charges, capitation, or some other methods for each specific type of benefit plan.

   ____

   ____

4. Do you use different fees and/or different methods for setting fees for different types of lab providers, e.g., physicians, hospital labs, independent labs? If so, discuss briefly. Do you have an additional payment for "STAT" tests? Do you pay for venipuncture (specimen collection)? If so, indicate the code used and any restrictions that may exist for payment.

5. What documentation do you require from laboratories for payment of claims?
(Please attach copies of lab claim forms)

6. If capitation rates are used for lab services, do they cover all tests in the CPT 80000 range or are some types of tests excluded? Do capitation rates for the lab include specimen collection in the physician's office and other specimen handling services? Do capitation rates to the lab differ by age, sex, or other member characteristics? Are risk corridors used for labs?

7. Please describe any other important characteristics of your payment methodology for laboratory tests.

Section II. Fee-for-Service Plans

Please provide in Table A, below, current fees paid (inclusive of patient copays) for the listed laboratory test codes under your benefit programs that pay for laboratory tests based on fee-for-service. Information on capitated payments for laboratory tests is requested in Section III. Provide fees for the following types of plans:

Indemnity
PPO
POS
HMO—private (nongovernment patients)
HMO—Medicare
HMO—Medicaid

If you use different fee schedules within one type of benefit plan (e.g., different fee schedules are used for two different HMO plans), provide the fees for the benefit plan with the largest enrollment. If you use different fee schedules for different markets, please make additional copies of Table A and provide data for each market area.

If different lab fees are used for different provider types (e.g., physicians, independent labs, and hospital labs), provide test fees for each and indicate how fees differ for other provider types (e.g., 10 percent higher for physicians than for independent labs).

If you use the same fee schedule for different types of plans (e.g., PPO and POS), provide the requested fee data for one plan and indicate with an asterisk that the same fees are used for the other plan(s).

TABLE A Laboratory Test Fees, 2000

CPT Code	Indemnity Plan	PPO Plan	POS Plan	HMO Plan (Private)	HMO (Medicare)	HMO (Medicaid)
*G0001	$	$	$	$	$	$
80049						
80054						
80061						
80092						
81000						
83036						
83970						
84153						
84154						
84443						
85024						
85025						
85610						
86316						
87086						
87536						
88142						
88164						
88305						
88307						
88342						

*G0001 (Medicare Code), or other code used for venipuncture–specimen collection.

Section III. Capitated Plans

For health benefit plans for which laboratory capitation is used, please provide in Table B, below, the monthly capitation rates (PMPM) used. Note, space is provided to list full or partial (some lab services excluded) laboratory capitation rates.

TABLE B PMPM Laboratory Test Capitation Rates, 2000

	POS Plan	HMO Plan (private)	HMO Plan (Medicare)	HMO Plan (Medicaid)
All Lab Services				
Partial Lab Services A*				
Partial Lab Services B**				

NOTE: * and ** indicate included and excluded services in the Additional Comments Section below.

Section IV. Additional Comments

Please provide any additional information that you believe will be helpful in our understanding of your laboratory payment methodologies.

____
____
____
____
____
____
____
____
____
____
____
____
____
____
____
____
____
____
____
____

APPENDIX D

Annual Volume of Laboratory Tests by Laboratory Type and Waived–Nonwaived Test Status, 1996–1998, 1999–Early 2000

TABLE D.1 Estimated Annual Volume of Laboratory Tests by Laboratory Type and Waived–Nonwaived[a] Test Status, 1996

Facility Type	Number of Laboratories	Waived Test Volume	Nonwaived Test Volume	Total Test Volume
Hospital	**8,888**	**91,883,111**	**2,886,279,172**	**2,978,162,283**
Independent	**5,751**	**15,886,008**	**1,529,300,443**	**1,545,166,451**
Physician				
Physician office	89,432	119,593,903	402,642,748	522,236,651
Community clinic	5,016	15,104,518	46,914,077	62,018,595
Health maintenance organization	959	6,879,396	58,602,448	65,481,844
Other practitioner	2,135	3,353,899	34,017,314	37,371,213
Total Physician	**97,542**	**144,931,716**	**542,176,587**	**687,108,303**
Other	11,216	64,978,527	235,688,932	300,667,459
Blood bank	338	9,037,496	108,378,714	117,416,210
Insurance	38	953,783	88,211,516	89,165,299
Ambulatory surgery center	1,160	1,892,906	24,881,423	26,774,329
Comp. outpatient rehabilitation facility	60	152,069	344,189	496,258
Ancillary test site in health facility	2,254	21,152,745	54,292,331	75,445,076

End-stage renal dialysis facility	1,919	7,034,302	3,698,366	10,732,668
Health fair	213	452,066	8,433,499	8,885,565
Home health agency	8,676	9,193,602	734,261	9,927,863
Hospice	596	377,998	2,020,628	2,398,626
Industrial	1,343	1,006,668	6,516,089	7,522,757
Intermediate care facility	626	419,097	1,570,654	1,989,751
Mobile unit	718	1,166,534	596,277	1,762,811
Pharmacy	288	150,911	142,638	293,549
School or student health service	1,175	1,072,946	3,797,719	4,870,665
Skilled nursing or nursing facility	13,933	37,638,543	5,968,203	43,606,746
Tissue bank	29	92,580	5,519,625	5,612,205
Rural health clinic or federally qualified health center[b]				
Ambulance[b]				
Total Other	**44,582**	**156,772,773**	**550,795,064**	**707,567,837**
Total, All Facility Types	**156,763**	**409,453,608**	**5,508,551,266**	**5,918,004,874**

[a]Tests are put in the waived category under (CLIA) regulations if they are simple to conduct, highly trained staff is not needed, and the chances for error are small. Facilities that conduct only waived tests do not have to meet the same personnel requirements as facilities that conduct moderate- or high-complexity tests.
[b]New facility types effective November 1998.

SOURCE: 1996 CLIA Provider Files. Health Care Financing Administration.

TABLE D.2 Estimated Annual Volume of Laboratory Tests by Laboratory Type and Waived–Nonwaived[a] Test Status, 1997

Facility Type	Number of Laboratories	Waived Test Volume	Nonwaived Test Volume	Total Test Volume
Hospital	**8,766**	**95,533,576**	**2,890,447,242**	**2,985,980,818**
Independent	**5,246**	**16,010,004**	**1,694,570,874**	**1,710,580,878**
Physician				
Physician office	91,979	125,431,118	531,817,599	657,248,717
Community clinic	5,667	16,507,804	56,348,445	72,856,249
Health maintenance organization	872	6,139,609	59,289,436	65,429,045
Other practitioner	2,113	3,087,842	38,034,249	41,122,091
Total Physician	**100,631**	**151,166,373**	**685,489,729**	**836,656,102**
Other	12,190	65,765,571	329,945,790	395,711,361
Blood bank	341	8,984,653	112,267,650	121,252,303
Insurance	36	953,348	106,422,639	107,375,987
Ambulatory surgery center	1,474	1,906,826	22,801,571	24,708,397
Comp. outpatient rehabilitation facility	86	120,763	313,722	434,485
Ancillary test site in health facility	2,629	22,165,830	57,195,905	79,361,735

End-stage renal dialysis facility	2,343	7,916,703	7,394,763	15,311,466
Health fair	262	536,936	8,229,977	8,766,913
Home health agency	11,202	10,594,655	759,040	11,353,695
Hospice	829	301,566	1,587,633	1,889,199
Industrial	1,375	993,481	19,482,917	20,476,398
Intermediate care facility	700	543,964	1,658,198	2,202,162
Mobile unit	1,074	1,403,132	2,871,039	4,274,171
Pharmacy	677	312,452	149,426	461,878
School or student health service	1,372	1,155,195	4,430,107	5,585,302
Skilled nursing or nursing facility	14,389	39,749,678	3,916,131	43,665,809
Tissue bank	33	93,830	5,492,474	5,586,304
Rural health clinic or federally qualified health center[b]				
Ambulance[b]				
Total Other	**51,012**	**163,498,583**	**684,918,982**	**848,417,565**
Total, All Facility Types	**165,655**	**426,208,536**	**5,955,426,827**	**6,381,635,363**

[a]Tests are put in the waived category under (CLIA) regulations if they are simple to conduct, highly trained staff is not needed, and the chances for error are small. Facilities that conduct only waived tests do not have to meet the same personnel requirements as facilities that conduct moderate- or high-complexity tests.
[b]New facility types effective November 1998.

SOURCE: 1997 CLIA Provider Files. Health Care Financing Administration.

TABLE D.3 Estimated Annual Volume of Laboratory Tests by Laboratory Type and Waived–Nonwaived[a] Test Status, 1998

Facility Type	Number of Laboratories	Waived Test Volume	Nonwaived Test Volume	Total Test Volume
Hospital	**8,644**	**94,196,474**	**2,861,419,809**	**2,955,616,283**
Independent	**4,871**	**15,272,621**	**1,380,135,459**	**1,395,408,080**
Physician				
Physician office	93,763	129,153,794	363,417,570	492,571,364
Community clinic	5,535	15,390,658	42,097,551	57,488,209
Health maintenance organization	751	5,042,666	30,487,001	35,529,667
Other practitioner	2,004	2,984,083	24,256,184	27,240,267
Total Physician	**102,053**	**152,571,201**	**460,258,306**	**612,829,507**
Other	11,995	64,685,709	217,678,933	282,364,642
Blood bank	316	8,595,502	96,113,181	104,708,683
Insurance	36	952,898	88,346,869	89,299,767
Ambulatory surgery center	1,507	1,933,819	20,287,811	22,221,630
Comp. outpatient rehabilitation facility	91	130,747	313,462	444,209
Ancillary test site in health facility	2,384	21,546,469	34,021,429	55,567,898

End-stage renal dialysis facility	2,386	7,742,580	5,875,977	13,618,557
Health fair	270	656,215	5,622,353	6,278,568
Home health agency	10,859	10,245,942	423,745	10,669,687
Hospice	847	305,926	1,415,242	1,721,168
Industrial	1,363	963,861	6,030,475	6,994,336
Intermediate care facility	665	520,100	624,787	1,144,887
Mobile unit	1,094	1,131,722	280,678	1,412,400
Pharmacy	773	447,319	110,149	557,468
School or student health service	1,379	1,214,093	3,648,558	4,862,651
Skilled nursing or nursing facility	14,008	38,971,818	3,006,791	41,978,609
Tissue bank	31	93,830	5,416,065	5,509,895
Rural health clinic or federally qualified health center[b]				
Ambulance[b]				
Total Other	**50,004**	**160,138,550**	**489,216,505**	**649,355,055**
Total, All Facility Types	**165,572**	**422,178,846**	**5,191,030,079**	**5,613,208,925**

[a]Tests are put in the waived category under (CLIA) regulations if they are simple to conduct, highly trained staff is not needed, and the chances for error are small. Facilities that conduct only waived tests do not have to meet the same personnel requirements as facilities that conduct moderate- or high-complexity tests.
[b]New facility types effective November 1998.

SOURCE: 1998 CLIA Provider Files. Health Care Financing Administration.

TABLE D.4 Estimated Annual Volume of Laboratory Tests by Laboratory Type and Waived–Nonwaived[a] Test Status, 1999–Early 2000

Facility Type	Number of Laboratories	Waived Test Volume	Nonwaived Test Volume	Total Test Volume
Hospital	**8,560**	**95,931,042**	**2,862,826,492**	**2,958,217,534**
Independent	**4,936**	**15,057,780**	**1,499,093,551**	**1,514,151,331**
Physician				
Physician office	96,357	133,563,773	347,739,610	481,303,383
Community clinic	5,978	18,360,107	40,200,559	58,560,666
Health maintenance organization	717	4,768,920	79,774,094	84,543,014
Other practitioner	2,037	3,350,368	28,679,024	32,029,392
Total Physician	**105,089**	**160,043,168**	**496,393,287**	**656,436,455**
Other	12,605	66,900	265,612,004	265,678,904
Blood bank	340	9,044,389	74,538,000	83,582,389
Insurance	44	961,946	79,440,076	80,402,022
Ambulatory surgery center	1,943	2,239,255	19,114,207	21,353,462
Comp. outpatient rehabilitation facility	107	317,250	450,541	767,791
Ancillary test site in health facility	2,650	22,437,640	4,116,747	26,554,387

End-stage renal dialysis facility	2,804	8,628,068	2,386,960	11,015,028
Health fair	315	501,270	12,732,801	13,234,071
Home health agency	8,461	17,570,371	326,868	17,897,239
Hospice	897	1,028,376	1,733,518	2,761,894
Industrial	1,428	954,110	6,224,404	7,178,514
Intermediate care facility	696	538,212	944,477	1,482,689
Mobile unit	1,203	1,663,769	2,140,582	3,804,351
Pharmacy	1,450	910,779	81,794	992,573
School or student health service	1,526	1,314,250	3,666,849	4,981,099
Skilled nursing or nursing facility	14,695	43,496,738	3,056,795	46,553,533
Tissue bank	41	99,930	7,633,868	7,733,798
Rural health clinic or federally qualified health center [b]	233	699,531	431,327	1,130,858
Ambulance [b]	79	20,360	-	20,360
Total Other	**51,517**	**112,493,144**	**484,631,818**	**597,124,962**
Total, All Facility Types	**170,102**	**382,985,134**	**5,342,945,148**	**5,725,930,282**

[a]Tests are put in the waived category under (CLIA) regulations if they are simple to conduct, highly trained staff is not needed, and the chances for error are small. Facilities that conduct only waived tests do not have to meet the same personnel requirements as facilities that conduct moderate- or high-complexity tests.
[b]New facility types effective November 1998.

SOURCE: March 2000 CLIA Provider Files. Health Care Financing Administration.

APPENDIX E

1998 Medicare Carrier Denial Rates

TABLE E.1 1998 Medicare Carrier Denial Rates for Top 100 CPT Codes

Obs. No.	CPT	Description	Total Claims	Allowed Services	Denied Claims	Percent Denied
1	G0001	Venipuncture	54,308,311	50,522,357	3,785,954	7
2	80061	Lipid panel	10,012,394	8,112,908	1,899,486	19
3	85025	Automated hemogram	13,484,091	10,641,281	2,842,810	21
4	84443	Assay TSH	5,871,658	4,579,775	1,291,883	22
5	80054	Comp metabolic panel	10,290,202	9,491,333	798,869	8
6	85024	Automated hemogram	8,662,269	7,358,832	1,303,437	15
7	84153	Assay of PSA, total	4,756,531	3,284,409	1,472,122	31
8	80092	Thyroid panel w/TSH	2,534,185	1,974,563	559,622	22
9	85610	Prothombin time	14,291,139	12,574,088	1,717,051	12
10	83036	Glycated hemoglobin test	5,066,357	4,162,652	903,705	18
11	80049	Metabolic panel, basic	5,828,554	5,468,084	360,470	6
12	81000	Urinalysis, nonauto w/scope	10,333,195	9,197,005	1,136,190	11
13	87086	Urine culture/colony count	3,470,828	2,977,871	492,957	14
14	83970	Assay of parathormone	607,387	563,481	43,906	7
15	88342	Immunocytochemistry	773,537	679,395	94,142	12
16	80162	Assay of digoxin	2,217,224	1,719,286	497,938	22
17	82607	Vitamin B-12	1,293,984	1,148,163	145,821	11
18	82728	Assay of ferritin	1,676,425	1,206,352	470,073	28
19	82947	Assay of glucose, quant	6,808,196	5,095,476	1,712,720	25
20	83718	Assay of lipoprotein	2,735,590	1,971,582	764,008	28
21	80058	Hepatic function panel	3,257,316	2,793,817	463,499	14
22	83550	Iron-binding test	2,222,641	1,672,426	550,215	25
23	83540	Assay of iron	3,125,180	2,065,183	1,059,997	34
24	85023	Automated hemogram	1,679,112	1,482,497	196,615	12
25	87186	Antibiotic sensitivity, mic	1,541,216	1,423,826	117,380	8
26	88312	Special stains	750,231	691,029	59,202	8
27	82746	Blood folic acid serum	912,478	791,881	120,597	13
28	80185	Assay of phenytoin, total	839,618	778,174	61,444	7

29	87340	Hep B surface antigen, EIA	1,066,065	990,005	76,060	7
30	82378	Carcinoembryonic antigen	717,046	523,034	194,012	27
31	88180	Cell marker study	765,834	578,032	187,802	25
32	87088	Urine bacteria culture	1,421,349	1,208,672	212,677	15
33	81001	Urinalysis, auto w/scope	3,123,900	2,832,521	291,379	9
34	82108	Assay of aluminum	374,227	347,575	26,652	7
35	83721	Assay of blood lipoprotein	1,016,926	890,414	126,512	12
36	85651	RBC sed rate, nonautomated	2,852,933	2,382,302	470,631	16
37	84439	Assay of free thyroxine	1,043,574	875,160	168,414	16
38	81002	Urinalysis nonauto w/o scope	3,672,390	3,040,808	631,582	17
39	84132	Assay of serum potassium	3,228,326	2,903,922	324,404	10
40	85027	Automated hemogram	1,347,928	1,117,113	230,815	17
41	80051	Electrolyte panel	1,686,997	1,564,619	122,378	7
42	84460	Alanine (alt) (SGPT)	4,473,439	4,022,030	451,409	10
43	82565	Assay of creatine	3,690,794	3,361,129	329,665	9
44	83735	Assay of magnesium	1,658,816	1,051,152	607,664	37
45	84436	Assay of total thyroxine	1,328,819	967,532	361,287	27
46	87070	Culture specimen, bacteria	795,903	732,725	63,178	8
47	88313	Special stains	714,671	644,559	70,112	10
48	82270	Test for blood, feces	3,582,984	2,406,732	1,176,252	33
49	84480	Assay, triiodothyronine (t^3)	478,533	427,966	50,567	11
50	86038	Antinuclear, antibodies	490,385	449,731	40,654	8
51	86235	Nuclear antigen antibodies	355,112	310,794	44,318	12
52	80059	Hepatitis panel	111,194	89,049	22,145	20
53	84165	Assay of serum proteins	478,051	441,159	36,892	8
54	82962	Glucose blood test	2,025,904	1,624,456	401,448	20
55	83615	Lactate (LD) (LDH) enzyme	3,590,958	3,229,463	361,495	10
56	82465	Assay of serum cholesterol	3,796,842	2,545,361	1,251,481	33
57	84550	Assay of blood uric acid	3,631,496	3,269,558	361,938	10
58	80164	Assay, dipropylaoctic acid	384,222	358,712	25,510	7
59	86316	Immunoassay, tumor antigen	380,049	230,267	149,782	39

Continued

TABLE E.1 *Continued*

Obs. No.	CPT	Description	Total Claims	Allowed Services	Denied Claims	Percent Denied
60	84520	Assay of urea nitrogen	3,142,103	2,829,708	312,395	10
61	84134	Assay of prealbumin	369,369	337,573	31,796	9
62	80091	Thyroid panel	494,986	341,512	153,474	31
63	87184	Antibiotic sensitivity, each	710,761	662,935	47,826	7
64	84466	Assay of transferrin	412,205	368,777	43,428	11
65	85021	Automated hemogram	945,869	785,785	160,084	17
66	88311	Decalcify tissues	521,382	476,714	44,668	9
67	84450	Transfarase (AST) (SGOT)	2,472,065	2,207,233	264,832	11
68	84403	Assay of total testosterone	182,640	166,282	16,358	9
69	80198	Assay of theophylline	316,372	296,049	20,323	6
70	85730	Thromboplastin time, partial	1,011,362	672,243	339,119	34
71	84100	Assay of phosphrus	3,277,539	2,945,742	331,797	10
72	88358	Analysis, tumor	45,022	33,684	11,338	25
73	82784	Assay of gammaglobulin IGM	475,411	443,826	31,585	7
74	80156	Assay of carbamazepine	290,031	270,482	19,549	7
75	87536	HIV-1 DNA, guant	61,753	50,847	10,906	18
76	88156	Cytopath cerv/vag tbs	1,123,563	705,034	418,529	37
77	p3000	Screen Pap by tech w md spuv		696,620		
78	86677	Helicobacter pylori	294,970	261,064	33,906	11
79	87163	Special microbiology culture	365,712	332,893	32,819	9
80	85022	Automated hemogram	721,987	625,796	96,191	13
81	86706	Hepatitis B surface antibody	318,970	291,801	27,169	9
82	82977	Assay of GGT	2,710,498	1,776,256	934,242	34
83	82985	Glycated protein	267,351	207,433	59,918	22
84	82310	Assay of calcium	1,835,714	1,627,676	208,038	11
85	84478	Assay of triglycerides	2,325,893	1,547,433	778,460	33
86	82150	Assay of amylase	522,595	457,640	64,955	12
87	81003	Urinalysis, auto w/o scope	1,524,186	1,304,784	219,402	14

88	80100	Drug screen	236,133	206,622	29,511	12
89	86803	Hepatitis c ab test	221,837	198,565	23,272	10
90	80101	Drug screen	281,363	242,105	39,258	14
91	82131	Amino acids, single quant	200,511	166,743	33,768	17
92	85045	Reticulocyte count	718,565	643,016	75,549	11
93	82550	Assay of CK (CPK)	992,983	888,071	104,912	11
94	88346	Immunofluorescent study	100,003	87,556	12,447	12
95	86003	Allergen specific ige	642,755	537,312	105,443	16
96	G0107	CA screen fecal blood test		909,427		
97	84295	Assay of serum sodium	1,605,560	1,449,005	156,555	10
98	86334	Immunofixation procedure	112,513	103,770	8,743	8
99	85007	Differential WBC Count	677,050	590,005	87,045	13
100	80158	Assay of cyclosporine	122,397	109,266	13,131	11
		AVERAGE	266,287,495	228,699,563	39,193,969	15

NOTE: The committee was unable to obtain an explanation for the denials. Since many of the tests with high denial rates are not screening tests, this does not fully explain the high denial rates. Other possible reasons for claims denials include stringent local medical review policies, contractors' inability to match ICD-9 codes with the appropriate CPT codes due to flaws in their computer programs, duplicative bills for a claim that was already paid, the patient is not eligible for benefits, the provider is not an approved Medicare provider, or the provider is billing for a type of test that is outside the laboratory's CLIA certification level. There appears to be no obvious pattern to the denial rates. One test that has a high rate of denial in one carrier region will have a very low denial rate in another carrier region.

AST = aspartate transominase; CK = creatine kinase; CPK = creatine phosphokinase; CPT = Current Procedural Terminology; EIA = enzyme immunoassay; GGT = γ-glutamyl transferase; MIC = minimum inhibitory concentration; PSA = prostate-specific antigen; RBC = red-blood cell; SGOT = serum glutamic–oxalvacetic transaminase; SGPT = serum glutamic–pyruvic transaminase; TSH = thyroid-stimulating hormone; WBC = white-blood cell.

TABLE E.2 1998 Medicare Carrier Denial Rates for the Top 20 Clinical Laboratory Tests, by State

		Denial Rate (percentage)								
		510	511	520	521	522	528	590	621	623
CPT Code	Description	AL	GA	AR	NM	OK	LA	FL	IL	MI
G0001	Venipuncture	5	7	5	8	6	7	7	7	5
80061	Lipid panel	14	17	5	25	14	16	15	23	17
85025	Automated hemogram	27	35	5	29	5	17	14	34	35
84443	Assay TSH	19	26	23	30	17	30	26	8	7
80054	Comp metabol panel	6	8	5	6	4	6	6	9	6
85024	Automated hemogram	18	16	4	6	8	13	12	19	19
84153	Assay of PSA, total[a]	41	33	53	32	11	50	41	29	30
80092	Thyroid panel w/TSH[b]	25	8	30	20	14	27	21	22	8
85610	Prothrombin time	9	12	4	14	12	12	13	15	15
83036	Glycated hemoglobin test	14	20	13	20	14	19	17	17	18
80049	Metabolic panel, basic	4	6	4	5	3	4	5	7	4
81000	Urinalysis, nonauto w/scope	20	16	13	7	12	5	8	9	6
87086	Urine culture/colony count	12	18	6	7	3	18	15	23	19
83970	Assay of parathormone	4	28	3	8	4	9	5	5	6
88342	Immunocytochemistry	21	6	12	33	25	12	10	31	21
80162	Assay of digoxin	30	49	26	17	12	22	24	47	53
82607	Vitamin B-12	5	6	6	6	3	8	6	9	6
82728	Assay of ferritin	32	33	53	38	17	55	9	15	17
82947	Assay of glucose, quant	25	27	21	14	8	19	29	26	39
83718	Assay of lipoprotein	19	27	7	45	29	37	34	40	41
80058	Hepatic function panel	48	46	6	5	4	47	5	7	4

Continued

TABLE E.2 *Continued*

		Denial Rate (percentage)								
		630	640	650	655	660	740	751	801	803
CPT Code	Description	IN	IA	KS	NE	KY	MO	MT	NY(W)	NY(E)
G0001	Venipuncture	7	4	2	3	5	4	32	7	12
80061	Lipid panel	15	9	23	25	15	34	19	7	20
85025	Automated hemogram	7	5	5	9	31	5	65	12	33
84443	Assay TSH	38	16	9	11	21	15	39	24	33
80054	Comp metabol panel	7	10	3	6	10	5	16	6	11
85024	Automated hemogram	9	7	3	6	14	4	29	6	27
84153	Assay of PSA, total[a]	54	46	30	30	26	36	41	46	46
80092	Thyroid panel w/TSH[b]	39	15	12	10	23	15	34	20	26
85610	Prothrombin time	16	2	7	6	43	9	34	12	21
83036	Glycated hemoglobin test	17	3	8	9	5	12	41	19	39
80049	Metabolic panel, basic	6	5	3	3	7	3	24	4	10
81000	Urinalysis, nonauto w/scope	6	13	4	5	12	7	38	14	22
87086	Urine culture/colony count	5	7	6	14	7	11	44	21	24
83970	Assay of parathormone	8	10	6	75	7	6	13	12	58
88342	Immunocytochemistry	7	11	5	8	23	7	1	7	10
80162	Assay of digoxin	17	2	12	12	7	13	33	21	30
82607	Vitamin B-12	10	42	3	5	8	4	43	18	20
82728	Assay of ferritin	49	19	24	23	33	26	62	42	46
82947	Assay of glucose, quant	12	9	17	16	27	20	22	43	41
83718	Assay of lipoprotein	17	14	46	40	17	34	68	34	28
80058	Hepatic function panel	6	4	3	4	15	4	15	4	9

Continued

TABLE E.2 *Continued*

CPT Code	Description	Denial Rate (percentage) 820 N/SD	824 CO	825 WY	831 AK	832 AZ	833 HI	834 NV	835 OR	836 WA	860 NJ
G0001	Venipuncture	4	10	7	4	12	4	10	5	6	4
80061	Lipid panel	8	23	15	16	33	7	26	14	6	29
85025	Automated hemogram	5	17	7	10	21	14	12	8	6	5
84443	Assay TSH	17	32	23	24	41	19	36	25	27	16
80054	Comp metabol panel	5	15	7	5	17	11	9	5	5	4
85024	Automated hemogram	7	8	9	15	6	10	6	12	7	6
84153	Assay of PSA, total[a]	53	54	46	36	33	20	35	26	27	21
80092	Thyroid panel w/TSH[b]	15	29	17	24	31	19	27	16	20	13
85610	Prothrombin time	5	14	9	10	24	13	24	10	14	10
83036	Glycated hemoglobin test	6	22	12	26	31	17	29	18	5	29
80049	Metabolic panel, basic	4	11	4	6	13	11	12	4	5	3
81000	Urinalysis, nonauto w/scope	12	25	15	7	9	10	21	8	7	10
87086	Urine culture/colony count	10	19	12	7	11	4	7	5	5	15
83970	Assay of parathormone	6	12	5	0	21	14	12	4	9	5
88342	Immunocytochemistry	5	12	11	40	14	5	3	4	9	8
80162	Assay of digoxin	1	13	7	4	15	4	8	4	5	20
82607	Vitamin B-12	50	57	49	3	20	4	11	6	6	5
82728	Assay of ferritin	24	46	39	28	47	17	38	24	32	46
82947	Assay of glucose, quant	10	24	12	22	48	26	44	28	10	25
83718	Assay of lipoprotein	12	42	23	33	36	18	36	23	7	19
80058	Hepatic function panel	5	10	6	19	66	9	75	24	5	4

Continued

TABLE E.2 *Continued*

		Denial Rate (percentage)									
		865	870	880	900	901	902	903	910	951	973
CPT Code	Description	PA	RI	SC	TX	MD	DE	DC	UT	WI	PR/VI
G0001	Venipuncture	4	15	6	5	6	18	5	7	4	6
80061	Lipid panel	20	16	34	13	13	19	27	25	13	7
85025	Automated hemogram	5	34	19	33	33	39	37	36	25	6
84443	Assay TSH	12	27	31	24	25	35	27	48	18	9
80054	Comp metabol panel	4	10	9	6	7	16	5	12	7	7
85024	Automated hemogram	5	8	25	18	21	5	14	24	21	5
84153	Assay of PSA, total[a]	18	35	61	21	27	36	31	27	24	23
80092	Thyroid panel w/TSH[b]	10	22	72	22	20	35	27	49	54	10
85610	Prothrombin time	6	20	17	15	15	16	18	15	12	6
83036	Glycated hemoglobin test	20	32	16	19	21	25	21	20	11	6
80049	Metabolic panel, basic	4	9	7	4	6	14	4	8	4	5
81000	Urinalysis, nonauto w/scope	6	8	9	7	10	18	9	7	4	6
87086	Urine culture/colony count	9	8	15	15	17	19	24	14	20	6
83970	Assay of parathormone	25	11	13	5	7	4	5	13	5	7
88342	Immunocytochemistry	5	28	12	4	3	1	5	5	4	12
80162	Assay of digoxin	15	9	34	23	24	38	31	17	19	4
82607	Vitamin B-12	4	12	9	9	8	38	5	20	39	5
82728	Assay of ferritin	26	45	30	30	33	47	34	59	21	6
82947	Assay of glucose, quant	15	19	30	22	33	41	39	34	9	23
83718	Assay of lipoprotein	21	28	46	24	19	42	30	36	19	15
80058	Hepatic function panel	3	8	8	5	7	9	4	9	4	7
G0001	Venipuncture	10	8	8	7	15	11	6	11	7	6
80061	Lipid panel	26	18	18	19	14	9	24	41	14	21

Continued

TABLE E.2 *Continued*

		Denial Rate (percentage)									
		2050	5130	5440	5535	10071	10230	10240	10250	10490	11260
CPT Code	Description	CA(T)	ID	TN	NC	RR	CT	MN	MS	VA	MO
85025	Automated hemogram	29	6	61	35	15	9	13	26	6	33
84443	Assay TSH	15	28	34	24	15	13	13	23	14	23
80054	Comp metabol panel	9	7	11	16	15	8	4	8	4	10
85024	Automated hemogram	19	8	32	31	16	9	40	26	7	22
84153	Assay of PSA, total[a]	25	40	32	44	15	7	52	34	18	46
80092	Thyroid panel w/TSH[b]	20	30	33	27	15	10	11		9	25
85610	Prothrombin time	7	14	14	12	15	7	7	17	8	13
83036	Glycated hemoglobin test	19	23	19	15	15	10	11	7	14	23
80049	Metabolic panel, basic	9	8	8	10	15	12	4	6	3	9
81000	Urinalysis, nonauto w/scope	15	7	11	17	16	13	18	21	13	7
87086	Urine culture/colony count	14	23	20	16	15	7	11	4	8	19
83970	Assay of parathormone	8	3	8	9	12	13	5	12	8	5
88342	Immunocytochemistry	14	8	12	11	24	14	16	12	11	27
80162	Assay of digoxin	9	13	20	27	15	8	12	16	7	16
82607	Vitamin B-12	11	5	11	38	16	11	3	12	7	5
82728	Assay of ferritin	31	42	16	38	13	44	10	20	8	30
82947	Assay of glucose, quant	20	38	29	30	19	13	4	24	18	41
83718	Assay of lipoprotein	16	30	28	20	19	14	21	22	9	25
80058	Hepatic function panel	11	5	9	9	14	10	4	6	4	53

Continued

TABLE E.2 *Continued*

		Denial Rate (percentage)							
		14330	16360	16510	31140	31142	31143	31144	31145
CPT Code	Description	NY(G)	OH	WV	CA(N)	ME	MA	NH	VT
G0001	Venipuncture	8	6	5	9	4	5	6	5
80061	Lipid panel	15	18	12	37	9	9	12	15
85025	Automated hemogram	24	7	6	12	9	7	11	10
84443	Assay TSH	16	24	16	47	16	15	19	22
80054	Comp metabol panel	7	7	5	14	6	5	10	4
85024	Automated hemogram	20	4	3	6	7	10	10	7
84153	Assay of PSA, total[a]	29	24	19	38	27	28	32	38
80092	Thyroid panel w/TSH[b]	16	40	37	44	14	10	16	11
85610	Prothrombin time	14	13	12	6	10	7	10	9
83036	Glycated hemoglobin test	14	15	10	10	14	11	16	22
80049	Metabolic panel, basic	4	5	4	8	3	4	5	5
81000	Urinalysis, nonauto w/scope	24	7	3	11	5	9	6	7
87086	Urine culture/colony count	16	14	8	6	17	11	18	16
83970	Assay of parathormone	8	15	4	3	10	5	7	NA
88342	Immunocytochemistry	12	4	3	10	5	11	4	2
80162	Assay of digoxin	17	24	22	7	21	15	19	25
82607	Vitamin B-12	13	7	6	1	8	6	10	4
82728	Assay of ferritin	41	33	27	5	29	19	22	30
82947	Assay of glucose, quant	44	22	15	15	19	25	28	19
83718	Assay of lipoprotein	14	27	20	56	16	21	21	19
80058	Hepatic function panel	6	5	4	69	5	4	7	5

Continued

TABLE E.2 *Continued*

NOTE: The committee was unable to obtain an explanation for the denials. Since many of the tests with high denial rates are not screening tests, this does not fully explain the high denial rates. Other possible reasons for claims denials include stringent local medical review policies, contractors' inability to match ICD-9 codes with the appropriate CPT codes due to flaws in their computer programs, duplicative bills for a claim that was already paid, the patient is not eligible for benefits, the provider is not an approved Medicare provider, or the provider is billing for a type of test that is outside the laboratory's CLIA certification level. There appears to be no obvious pattern to the denial rates. One test that has a high rate of denial in one carrier region will have a very low denial rate in another carrier region.

LMRP = local medical review policy; PSA = prostate specific antigen; TSH = thyroid-stimulating hormone.

[a]Coverage was recently extended to screening, once per year.
[b]Panel was eliminated in 2000 but there will still be LMRP for each individual test.

APPENDIX F

Committee Biographies

Lauren LeRoy, Ph.D., is president and chief executive officer of Grantmakers In Health, a nonprofit educational organization serving health foundations. Previously, she was executive director of the Medicare Payment Advisory Commission (MedPAC), a nonpartisan congressional advisory body. Prior to MedPAC, she served as executive director of the Physician Payment Review Commission (PPRC). She came to PPRC from the Commonwealth Fund Commission on Elderly People Living Alone, where she served as associate director. Dr. LeRoy spent more than a decade at the Institute for Health Policy Studies, University of California, San Francisco, where she was assistant director and directed the Institute's Washington office. She began her career as a health policy analyst in the Department of Health, Education, and Welfare. Dr. LeRoy's work has focused on Medicare reform, the health work force, health care for the elderly, and health philanthropy. She received a doctorate in social policy planning from the University of California, Berkeley. She is a member of the National Academy of Social Insurance and a fellow of the Academy for Health Services Research and Health Policy.

Howard Bailit, D.M.D., Ph.D., is professor and director of the Health Policy and Primary Care Research Center at the University of Connecticut School of Medicine and a research associate at the Sloan Managed Care Research Center, Harvard University. He is responsible for developing health services and policy research at the University of Connecticut. Prior to these positions, he was a senior vice president for medical policy and programs at Aetna Health Plans (1986–1995). He has also held academic positions at Columbia University, School of Public Health (1982–1986), where he chaired the Department of

Health Administration and Policy, and the University of Connecticut Health Center (1967–1982), where he served as head of Behavioral Sciences and Community Health. He received his dental degree from Tufts and his Ph.D. from Harvard. He has published widely on health policy and managed care and serves on many national committees and editorial boards. He has been a member of the Institute of Medicine (IOM) since 1984.

Christopher Bladen, M.Sc., has more than five years' experience as an independent consultant. His activities have chiefly been devoted to providing advice to donor agencies, developing countries, and newly independent nations of the former Soviet Bloc regarding health care and health care financing reform, and conducting baseline studies of health sector costs. For 20 years, Mr. Bladen served in the health policy component of the Office of the Assistant Secretary for Planning and Evaluation, U.S. Department of Health and Human Services (DHHS). During this period he directed the Divisions of Science and Health Policy, Health Care Financing, and Health Economics. Prior to his retirement, he served as the deputy to the deputy assistant secretary for health policy for five years. He received his B.A. (political science) from Williams College, Williamstown, Massachusetts, and his M.Sc. (economics) from the London School of Economics and Political Science, London, UK; he passed Ph.D. comprehensive examinations (political science) from the Maxwell School, Syracuse University, Syracuse, N.Y. Mr. Bladen has received a postdoctoral fellowship from the American Society for Public Administration. He has also received various departmental and secretarial awards from the U.S. Departments of Commerce and Health and Human Services.

William Hsiao, Ph.D., is the K.T. Li Professor of Economics and director of the Program in Health Care Financing at the Harvard School of Public Health. His current research focuses on developing a theory of health system economics. His research also concentrates on payment for hospital and physician services, social and private insurance, and competition in managed care markets. Dr. Hsiao received his Ph.D. in economics from Harvard University, and he is also a qualified actuary. He was named the Man of the Year in Medicine for his work developing a rational fee schedule for physician services, the resource-based relative value scale (RBRVS), which has been adopted by the United States, Australia, Canada, and France. He was awarded honorary professorships by several leading Chinese universities. He is a member of the National Academy of Sciences and serves on the Board of Directors for both the National Academy of Social Insurance and the Society of Actuaries. He has advised the U.S. Congress, the White House, the World Bank, the International Monetary Fund, the World Health Organization, and many nations.

William B. Kerr, M.H.A., is currently the Senior Vice President of The Hunter Group. He served in a variety of administrative positions at the University of California, San Francisco Medical Center over the past 30 years, including 19 years as medical center director. Mr. Kerr earned a B.S. in social science from Loyola University in 1964 and a graduate degree in hospital administration from the University of Minnesota in 1969. He was the recipient of the California Association of Hospitals and Health Systems Certificate of Distinction, the Association of American Medical Colleges Distinguished Service Award, and the University of California San Francisco Medal. Mr. Kerr served as a member of the Board of Governors of the National Institutes of Health Clinical Center and is currently a member of the IOM and the Commonwealth Fund Task Force on Academic Health Centers.

J. Stephen Kroger, M.D., is Chief Executive Officer of COLA (formerly the Commission on Office Laboratory Accreditation), an organization that accredits more than 7,200 physician office laboratories in the United States. His past experience includes 25 years of direct patient care as a practicing internist, development of workable standards for office laboratories, implementation of the Clinical Laboratory Improvement Amendments regulations, and work in the general areas of quality improvement in the laboratory and medical practice settings. He has served as a consultant to the Centers for Disease Control and Prevention, and served as a member of the DHHS Clinical Laboratory Improvement Advisory Committee from 1992 to 1996. He has testified before various House and Senate subcommittees on laboratory issues. He is a fellow of the American College of Physicians and a member of the American Medical Association and the American Society of Association Executives. Dr. Kroger received his doctorate in medicine from the University of Cincinnati in 1965 and board certification in internal medicine in 1972.

John Matsen, M.D., is a Professor Emeritus of pathology and pediatrics at the University of Utah. He served as chair of the Department of Pathology from 1981 to 1993. He was the president and chief executive officer of Associated Regional and University Pathologists, Inc. from 1984 to 1993 and board chair from 1993 to 1999. Dr. Matsen served as senior vice president for health sciences at the University of Utah from January 1993 to December 1998. He has served as president of the Academy of Clinical Laboratory Physicians and Scientists and as president of the Association of Pathology Chairs. Dr. Matsen's M.D. degree was awarded by the University of California at Los Angeles. He is the recipient of many prestigious awards including the Becton-Dickinson Award from the American Society for Microbiology. Dr. Matsen currently serves on the Board of Directors of ASM-Resources, Inc., a for-profit, subsidiary corporation of the American Society for Microbiology.

Stephen T. Mennemeyer, Ph.D., is a professor in the Department of Health Care Organization and Policy, School of Public Health, University of Alabama at Birmingham. He teaches and conducts research on health economics and the cost-effectiveness of health care interventions. Previously he was senior economist at Abt Associates Inc. in Cambridge, Massachusetts. There he conducted studies of the administrative costs of the Medicare program, competitive bidding systems, and patient outcomes following clinical laboratory tests. Dr. Mennemeyer holds a Ph.D. in economics from the State University of New York at Buffalo. He is a member of the American Economics Association, American Public Health Association, International Health Economics Association, Society for Medical Decision Making, and Southern Economics Association.

David L. Smalley, Ph.D., is a professor of pathology at the University of Tennessee, Health Sciences Center, Memphis, Tennessee. He has been a faculty member with the University since 1980 and has been actively involved in teaching and research at the medical school, allied health programs, and residency programs. He also serves as technical director of the Memphis Pathology Laboratory (MPL), L.L.C. in Memphis. Dr. Smalley has been a consultant to MPL since 1986, serving as the technical director for immunology and clinical chemistry. Dr. Smalley holds a bachelor's degree in medical technology. He holds a master's degree and Ph.D. in microbiology–immunology and is licensed by the State of Tennessee as a general medical laboratory director. He was the 1998 recipient of the Outstanding Reserve/Guard Laboratorian Award from the Society for Armed Forces Medical Laboratory Scientists. He is a member of the American Association of Bioanalysts, American Society for Microbiology, Clinical Laboratory Management Association, and American Association of Immunologists.

Earl P. Steinberg, M.D., M.P.P., is a senior vice president of research and development and industry affairs for Resolution Health Strategies, Inc. and an adjunct professor of medicine and of health policy and management at Johns Hopkins University. From 1994 to February 2000, Dr. Steinberg was vice president of Covance Health Economics and Outcomes Services Inc., director of its Quality Assessment and Improvement Systems Division, and codirector of its Outcomes Studies Group. Prior to joining Covance, Dr. Steinberg was professor of medicine and of health policy and management at Johns Hopkins University, and director of the Johns Hopkins Program for Medical Technology and Practice Assessment. While at Johns Hopkins, Dr. Steinberg was the principal investigator on the federally funded Patient Outcome Research Team that evaluated the management of cataracts. Dr. Steinberg received his A.B. degree from Harvard College (summa cum laude), his M.D. from Harvard Medical School, and a master of public policy degree from the Kennedy School of Government at Harvard. His residency training in internal medicine was performed at the Massachusetts General Hospital. Dr. Steinberg has received numerous awards and is a fellow of the American College of Physicians and the Academy for Health Services Research and Health Policy. He has served for 10 years as a member of the National Blue Cross/Blue Shield Association's Medical Advisory Panel and served for four years on the federal Physician Payment Review Commission.

Bruce Steinwald, M.B.A., is an independent consultant in Washington, D.C., specializing in health economics consulting for health care delivery and financing organizations. Until the fall of 1999, Mr. Steinwald was a senior fellow at the National Health Policy Forum, George Washington University, and before that he was vice president of Covance Health Economics and Outcomes Services, Inc. where he directed the company's Outcomes Studies Group and initiated its European practice. In the 1980s, Mr. Steinwald worked in the Office of the Secretary, Department of Health and Human Services, and was deputy director of the Prospective Payment Assessment Commission (now MedPAC). He received his B.A. degree from Johns Hopkins University and his M.B.A. in health administration from the University of Chicago, Graduate School of Business, where he also completed all requirements except the dissertation for a Ph.D. in economics. Mr. Steinwald served on the National Committee on Vital and Health Statistics from 1988 to 1996 and is currently a member of the Academy for Health Services Research and Health Policy and the Society for Health Service Administrators.

Eleanor Travers, M.D., M.H.A., is a physician executive and health care system administrator, currently in public service at the U.S. Department of Veterans Affairs (VA) Headquarters in Washington, D.C, where she is the clinical manager for utilization and capacity management and the national medical advisor for cost-effectiveness. Previously, she was a chief executive officer and medical director for the nation's largest clinical laboratory system and chief of service and professor at numerous medical school-affiliated hospitals. Dr. Travers has a wide scope of health care administrative, legislative policy, quality, and cost analysis experience and is nationally known for her textbooks, published writings, and teaching on laboratory management and cost accounting. She created the legislative pathway for and authored the VA's Clinical Laboratory Improvement Amendments in 1993 and has testified before the Congress as an expert in quality improvement, personnel, and information technology issues. From 1984 to 1987 she served on the Methods Panel for the IOM Council on Health Care Technology. She is a graduate of Boston University (AB), the Medical College of Pennsylvania (MD), and George Washington University (MHA).